The Anesthesia Drug Handbook

NOTICE

Every effort has been made to ensure that the drug dosage schedules herein are accurate and in accord with the standards accepted at the time of publication. However, as new research and experience broaden our knowledge, changes in treatment and drug therapy occur. The medications described do not necessarily have specific approval by the Food and Drug Administration for use in the situations and dosages for which they are recommended. This information is advisory only. The package insert should be consulted for use and dosage as approved by the FDA for any changes in indications and dosages and for added warnings and precautions. The ultimate responsibility lies with the prescribing physician.

The Anesthesia Drug Handbook

SOTA OMOIGUI, M.D.
Assistant Professor of Anesthesiology
Department of Anesthesiology
Charles R. Drew University of Medicine and
 Science
Attending Anesthesiologist
King/Drew Medical Center
Los Angeles, California

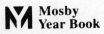
Mosby
Year Book

St. Louis   Baltimore   Boston   Chicago   London   Philadelphia   Sydney   Toronto

CONSULTING EDITORS

Louis Alexander, M.D.
Attending Anesthesiologist
Cook County Hospital
Chicago, Illinois

Nowa Omoigui, M.D., M.P.H.
Fellow, Division of Cardiovascular Medicine
Stanford University School of Medicine
Falk Cardiovascular Research Center
Stanford, California

Julie Pippins, Pharm.D.
Clinical Coordinator
Pharmacy Services
Veterans Administration Hospital
Shreveport, Louisiana

Shirley Randall, M.D.
Attending Anesthesiologist
Womack Army Hospital
Fayetteville, North Carolina

John Stewart, Ph.D.
Professor of Pharmacology
Louisiana State University Medical Center
Shreveport, Louisiana

Mosby
Year Book

Dedicated to Publishing Excellence

Sponsoring Editor: Susan M. Gay
Associate Managing Editor, Manuscript Services: Deborah Thorp
Production Manager: Nancy C. Baker
Proofroom Manager: Barbara Kelly

1 2 3 4 5 6 7 8 9 0 CL/ML 96 95 94 93 92

Library of Congress Cataloging-in-Publication Data
Omoigui, Sota.
    Anesthesia drug handbook / Sota Omoigui.
        p.   cm.
    Includes bibliographical references and index.
    ISBN 0–8016–6898–0
    1. Anesthetics—Handbooks, manuals, etc. 2. Anesthesia adjuvants—
-Handbooks, manuals, etc.   3. Pharmacology—Handbooks, manuals, etc.
I. Title.
    [DNLM: 1. Anesthesia—handbooks.   2. Anesthetics—handbooks.
3. Drug Interactions—handbooks.   WO 231 056a]
RD85.5.046 1992   92–12908
617.9′6—dc20   CIP
DNLM/DLC
for Library of Congress

FOREWORD

Anesthesiology is a specialty that requires extensive medical knowledge, particularly in pharmacology. A competent anesthesiologist is expected to be familiar not only with all the drugs he or she prescribes and uses in the course of care, but also those drugs prescribed by other specialists with whom the modern-day anesthesiologist must interact. Anesthetic techniques have progressed from the relatively simple open-drop ether method to balanced multiple-drug manipulations utilizing a variety of intravenous and inhalational agents.

There are several classic reference textbooks of pharmacology. They tend to remain on bookshelves as daunting evidence of the vast knowledge required of contemporary physicians. There has long been a need for a concise pocket-book readily available during preoperative visits, in the operating room, and in the intensive care unit. The publication of this *Anesthesia Drug Handbook* is, therefore, welcome and timely.

It is a remarkably comprehensive pocket-sized manual of drugs and anesthetic agents used or commonly encountered by anesthesiologists. All of the drugs are listed in alphabetical order, making rapid retrieval of information possible. Each drug is presented in a consistent style, with information on uses (indications), dosing, elimination, how supplied, pharmacology, pharmocokinetics, guidelines/precautions, and principal adverse reactions.

It is written in three parts. Part I includes almost all of the intravenous drugs used in the operating room and the intensive care unit. Part II includes all inhalational anesthetics. Part III, which contains the appendixes includes malignant hyperthermia protocol, cardiopulmonary resuscitation algorithms, and infusion tables of all intravenous drugs listed in the text.

Dr. Omoigui has clearly demonstrated sensitivity to the demands of frontline anesthesia in writing this book. I commend it, therefore, as an invaluable addition to the armamentarium of all anesthesiologists, in training and in practice.

Fun Sun Yao, M.D.
Associate Professor of Anesthesiology
Cornell Medical College
Attending Anesthesiologist
The New York Hospital
New York, New York

Note: *This publication is available from Med-Pharm Information Systems (618 242-4934) or Mosby Yearbook Publishers (800 325-4177) in a software format for the IBM PC and compatibles. For on-site retrieval of information, the software may be licensed for use in critical care unit terminals, anesthesia machines or compatible patient monitoring systems. Manufacturers of patient monitors and information terminals should obtain licenses from Med-Pharm Information Systems. (608 N 12th Street, Mount Vernon, Illinois.)*

PREFACE

The large and rapidly expanding field of anesthetic pharmacology has witnessed a dramatic proliferation of drugs available to the anesthesiologist. These drugs are administered as boluses or infusions by various routes, such as intravenous, sublingual, oral, rectal, intranasal, intrapleural, transdermal, intraarticular, inhalational, epidural, caudal, and spinal.

The current state of the art requires an intimate familiarity with dosing information and pharmacology for this plethora of new drugs, and new indications/routes of administration for old drugs. This may be overwhelming, not only to the trainee but also to the seasoned practitioner. The urgency of decision making in the operating rooms or critical care units allows little room for error; there is a need for this pocket-sized compendium that enables the anesthesiologist to identify a drug, its dose, route of administration, and side effects at a moment's notice.

The *Anesthesia Drug Handbook* reviews basic fundamentals of pharmacology and profiles the drugs and inhalational agents commonly used in anesthesia. Rather than providing a comprehensive description, the focus is on selected information required for proper use of each drug. The use of this drug handbook requires a well-founded basic knowledge and practical experience that is essential for patient safety.

This handbook has been designed to fit the pocket of your operating room gown or scrub suit. It is hoped that it will make the difference in providing optimal patient care.

Sota Omoigui, M.D.

ACKNOWLEDGMENTS

The completion of this work has been made possible by the time and effort of many people. Special thanks to Carletta Brown at Duke University for her endless patience in the preparation of the manuscript; Agaytha Stewart at Med-Pharm Information Systems for assistance in the electronic publication; Russel Carpenter at Micro-Age Computers for computer support; Susan Gay and Lauranne Billus at Mosby–Year Book for their editorial support; Didaciane Gatete for preparation of the infusion tables; and the consulting editors for a meticulous and painstaking review. Finally, I wish to acknowledge Professors Jerry Reves and Antonio Aldrete, whose contributions to the specialty are an inspiration to the younger generation of anesthesiologists.

Sota Omoigui, M.D.

CONTENTS

DRUGS

ADENOSINE (ADENOCARD)

Use(s): Treatment of acute paroxysmal supraventricular tachycardia (PSVT); differentiation of supraventricular tachycardia with intraventricular aberrancy from ventricular tachycardia; controlled hypotension during cerebral aneurysm surgery; pharmacologic stress testing (e.g., with thallium) in coronary artery disease.

Dosing: Treatment/diagnosis of PSVT: Rapid IV bolus: 6–12 mg (children, 0.05–0.25 mg/kg). May be repeated within 1–2 min (for two doses) if necessary. Single doses > 12 mg are not recommended. More effective when administered via a central vein or into the right atrium.

Elimination: Cellular uptake and metabolism (deamination, phosphorylation).

How Supplied: Injection, 3 mg/mL.

Pharmacology

An endogenous nucleoside with antiarrythmic activity, adenosine slows conduction through the A-V node. It can interrupt the reentry pathways through the A-V node and restore normal sinus rhythm in patients with acute PSVT, including that associated with Wolff-Parkinson-White syndrome. It decreases peripheral resistance and arterial pressure. Unlike verapamil, systemic hemodynamic effects are minimal and transient. The electrophysiologic effects of adenosine are not blocked by atropine, which indicates a lack of vagal mediation. Adenosine does not convert atrial flutter, atrial fibrillation, or ventricular tachycardia to normal sinus rhythm (with the rare exception of adenosine-sensitive ventricular tachycardia). Modest slowing of ventricular response may occur with atrial flutter or fibrillation.

Pharmacokinetics

Onset: <20 sec
Peak effect: 20–30 sec
Duration: 3–7 sec
Interaction/toxicity: Prolonged bradycardia in patients with toxic concentrations of calcium channel blockers; antagonized competitively by methylxanthines, e.g., theophylline or caffeine; potentiated by blockers of nucleoside transport, e.g., dipyridamole; increased heart rate with nicotine; higher degrees of heart block in the presence of carbamazepine.

Guidelines/Precautions

1. Do not confuse this drug with adenosine phosphate, which is used as adjunctive therapy in the treatment of complications associated with varicose veins.
2. Due to the rapid metabolism, it is imperative to administer the dose rapidly over 2–3 sec. If given at a slower rate, a reflex tachycardia may occur as a result of systemic vasodilation. Negative chronotropic and dromotropic effects are only seen with rapid administration.
3. Adenosine may produce a short-lasting first-, second-, or third-degree heart block. Do not give additional doses if patients develop a high-level block.
4. It is not effective in patients receiving methylxanthines which, can completely block the electrophysiologic effects.
5. Use with caution in patients capable of rapid A-V conduction. Atrial fibrillation or flutter have been observed in patients receiving adenosine.
6. Reduce doses in heart transplant patients. Donor sinus and A-V nodes may have increased response to adenosine compared with recipient nodes or control subjects.
7. Significantly lower doses of adenosine should be administered in patients receiving dipyridamole. Initial doses should not exceed 1 mg.
8. Use with caution in patients with asthma. It may cause bronchoconstriction.

9. ECG monitoring is essential to determine conversion to normal sinus rhythm or A-V block and detect arrhythmias.
10. Contraindicated in patients with second- or third-degree A-V block or sick sinus syndrome, except cases in which a pacemaker has been placed.

Principal Adverse Reactions

Cardiovascular: Palpitations, chest pain, hypotension, bradycardia, arrhythmias.
Pulmonary: Dyspnea, hyperventilation.
CNS: Headache, dizziness, blurred vision, numbness, irritability.
GI: Nausea, metallic taste, tightness in throat.
Dermatologic: Flushing.

ALFENTANIL HCL (ALFENTA)

Use(s): Analgesia, anesthesia.
Dosing: : Analgesia: IV/IM, 10–25 μg/kg.
    Induction: IV, 50–150 μg/kg.
    Infusion: 0.1–3 μg/kg/min.
    Epidural: Bolus, 10–20 μg/kg; infusion, 100–250 μg/hr.
Elimination: Hepatic.
How Supplied: Injection, 500 μg/mL.
Dilution for Infusion: IV, 10 mg (20 mL) alfentanil in 250 mL of D5W or normal saline (NS) solution (40 μg/mL); epidural, 1.5 mg (3 mL) alfentanil in 150 mL local anesthetic or (preservative free) NS solution (10 μg/mL).

Pharmacology

A potent opioid analgesic with rapid onset and short duration of action. Alfentanil produces a deep level of analgesia and attenuates the hemodynamic response to surgical stress. Like most opiods, it may also produce bradycardia, especially in conjunction with nonvagolytic neuromuscular blocking agents (e.g., vecuronium) or in the absence of an anticholinergic drug. Induction doses produce respiratory depression and decreases in blood pressure secondary to peripheral vasodilation. Alfentanil is associated with more hypotension and bradycardia than either fentanyl or sufentanil. Repeated doses or continuous infusions do not result in a significant cumulation.

Pharmacokinetics

Onset: IV, 1–2 min; IM, <5 min; epidural, 5–15 min.
Peak Effect: IV, 1–2 min; IM, <15 min; epidural, 30 min.
Duration: IV, 10–15 min; IM, 10–60 min; epidural, 4–8 hr.
Interaction/Toxicity: Circulatory and ventilatory depressant effects potentiated by narcotics, sedatives, volatile anesthetics, nitrous oxide; ventilatory depressant effects potentiated by amphetamines, monoamine oxidase (MAO) inhibitors, phenothiazines, and tricyclic antidepressants; analgesia enhanced by α_2-agonists, e.g., clonidine, epinephrine; reduced clearance and prolonged respiratory depression with concomitant use of erythromycin; muscle rigidity in higher dose range sufficient to interfere with ventilation.

Guidelines/Precautions

1. Reduce doses in elderly, hypovolemic, high-risk surgical patients and with concomitant use of sedatives and other narcotics.
2. Narcotic effects reversed by naloxone (≥0.2–0.4 mg IV).
3. Excessive bradycardia may be treated with atropine.
4. Crosses the placental barrier, and usage in labor may produce depression of respiration in the neonate. Resuscitation may be required; have naloxone available.
5. Epidural alfentanil (all epidural, caudal, or intrathecal narcotics) may cause delayed respiratory depression (up to 8 hr after single dose of alfentanil, fentanyl, sufentanil; up to 24 hours for morphine), pruritus, nausea, and vomiting, urinary retention. Naloxone (0.2–0.4 mg IV prn or infusion 5–10 µg/kg/hr) is effective for prophylaxis and/or treatment. Ventilatory support for respiratory depression must be readily available. Antihistamines, e.g., diphenhydramine (12.5–25 mg IV/IM q6h prn), may be used for pruritus. Metoclopramide (10 mg IV q6h prn) may be used for nausea and vomiting. Urinary retention may require straight bladder catheterization.
6. Epidural/intrathecal injections should be avoided when the

patient has septicemia, infection at the injection site, or coagulopathy.

Principal Adverse Reactions

Cardiovascular: Bradycardia, hypotension, arrhythmias.
Pulmonary: Respiratory depression.
CNS: Euphoria, dysphoria, convulsions.
GI: Nausea and vomiting, biliary tract spasm, delayed gastric emptying.
Musculoskeletal: Muscle rigidity.
Other: Pruritus.

AMINOCAPROIC ACID (AMICAR)

Use(s): Treatment of life-threatening bleeding disorders secondary to systemic hyperfibrinolysis or urinary fibrinolysis; prophylaxis against recurrent subarachnoid hemorrhage.
Dosing: IV/PO, 4–5 g in 1 hr, then IV/PO, 1–1.25 g/hr. Continue for about 8 hr or until bleeding is controlled.
Elimination: Renal.
How Supplied: Injection, 250 mg/mL; tablets, 500 mg; oral solution, 250 mg/mL.
Dilution for Infusion: 15 g in 500 mL NS solution (30 mg/mL).

Pharmacology

As an inhibitor of plasminogen activators and, to a lesser extent, plasmin, this drug is useful in enhancing hemostasis when fibrinolysis contributes to bleeding. In life-threatening situations, fresh whole blood transfusions, fibrinogen infusions, and other emergency measures may be required. Aminocaproic acid should not be used without heparin when there is evidence of active intravascular coagulation.

Pharmacokinetics

Onset: IV, almost immediate; PO, few minutes.
Peak Effect: IV, 1–3 hr; PO, <2 hr.
Duration: IV/PO, 3–5 hr.
Interaction/Toxicity: Hypotension, bradycardia, arrhythmia from

rapid IV injection; serious or fatal thrombus formation in disseminated intravascular coagulation.

Guidelines/Precautions

1. Do not use without a definitive diagnosis of hyperfibrinolysis.
2. Increased risk of hypercoagulability in patients taking estrogens or estrogen-containing oral contraceptives.
3. Injectable form not for use in newborns because of toxicity of preservative (benzyl alcohol).

Principal Adverse Reactions

Cardiovascular: Hypotension, bradycardia.
CNS: Dizziness, tinnitus.
GI: Nausea, cramps, diarrhea.
Musculoskeletal: Myopathy, rhabdomyolysis.
GU: Renal failure.

AMINOPHYLLINE (AMINOPHYLLINE)

Use(s): Prevention and treatment of bronchial asthma and reversal of bronchospasm associated with chronic obstructive pulmonary disease.

Dosing: Loading: IV, 5–6 mg/kg (give over 20–30 min) or PO/rectal, 6 mg/kg. Each 0.5 mg/kg theophylline (0.6 mg/kg aminophylline) will increase theophylline concentration by 1 µg/mL.

Maintenance: IV, 0.5–1 mg/kg/hr; PO, 2–4 mg/kg q6–12h.

Lower end of dose range should be used with infants, older patients, patients with cor pulmonale or congestive heart failure (CHF) and those receiving theophylline. Higher end of dose range should be used with children and young adult smokers. Therapeutic level: 10–20 µg/mL.

Elimination: Hepatic.

How Supplied: Injection, 1 mg/mL, 2 mg/mL, 25 mg/mL; tablets, 100 mg, 200 mg; tablets (sustained release), 225 mg; oral solution, 105 mg/5 mL; rectal solution, 60 mg/mL; rectal suppositories, 250 mg, 500 mg. 100 mg of aminophylline is equivalent to 78.9 mg anhydrous theophylline.

Dilution for Infusion: Loading dose: dilute in 50 mL D_5W or NS. Maintenance dose: dilute 500 mg in 500 mL D_5W or NS (1 mg/mL).

Pharmacology

Aminophylline is converted to theophylline. The exact mechanism of action is unclear. Theophylline, a methylxanthine bronchodilator, may produce its pharmacologic effects by inhibiting phosphodiesterase, thereby increasing the levels of cyclic adenosine monophosphate (cAMP) in bronchial smooth muscle; by blocking adenosine receptors; antagonism of prostaglandin E_2; or a direct effect on the mobilization of calcium. It reduces fatigue of diaphragmatic muscles, increases cardiac output, and decreases peripheral vascular resistance.

Pharmacokinetics

Onset: IV, few minutes; PO, within 30 min.
Peak Effect: IV, 1 hr; PO, 1–2 hr.
Duration: PO, 4–8 hr.
Interaction/Toxicity: Elevated serum levels in patients receiving cimetidine, β-blockers, allopurinol, oral contraceptive corticosteroids, quinolone antibiotics, e.g., norfloxacin, macrolide antibiotics, e.g., erythromycin, and in patients with cardiac failure, liver insufficiency; decreased serum levels with phenobarbital, phenytoin, rifampin, and smokers; aminophylline antagonizes effects of propranolol, potentiates pressor effects of sympathomimetics, and may produce seizures, cardiac arrhythmias, cardiorespiratory arrest, ventricular arrhythmia with excessive plasma levels, or in patients receiving volatile anesthetics, especially halothane.

Guidelines/Precautions

1. Frequent monitoring of plasma concentrations. Increased toxicity at serum concentration >20 μg/mL. Treatment of toxicity includes cessation of therapy and supportive and symptomatic treatment.
2. Avoid rapid infusions. May cause hypotension, arrhythmias, and possibly death.
3. Wait 3 drug half-lives after the last dose of aminophylline is

given (i.e., approximately 13 hr in normal individuals) before using halothane to anesthetize an asthmatic patient. Use isoflurane or enflurane in patients who must be given aminophylline or other exogenous sympathomimetic drugs before or during surgery.

Principal Adverse Reactions

Cardiovascular: Palpitation, sinus tachycardia, supraventricular and ventricular arrhythmias.
Pulmonary: Tachypnea.
CNS: Seizures, headache, irritability.
GI: Nausea, vomiting, epigastric pain.
Other: Hyperglycemia, syndrome of inappropriate antidiuretic hormone (SIADH).

AMIODARONE (CORDARONE)

Use(s): Treatment of life-threatening ventricular arrhythmias that do not respond to other antiarrhythmics; selective treatment of supraventricular tachyarrhythmias.
Dosing: PO loading: 800–1600 mg/day for 1–3 wk.
PO maintenance: 200–600 mg/day.
Therapeutic level: 1.0–2.5 μg/mL.
Elimination: Hepatic.
How Supplied: Tablets, 200 mg; injection, not approved for general clinical use in the United States.

Pharmacology

This benzofuran derivative has mixed class 1C and III antiarrhythmic characteristics. It (1) prolongs action potential duration and increases the refractory period of cardiac fibers, including accessory pathways; (2) causes noncompetitive alpha- and beta-adrenergic inhibition. Long-term therapy results in dilation of coronary arteries and increased coronary blood flow.

Pharmacokinetics

Onset: 2–4 days but may be delayed much longer (e.g., 2–3 mo).

Peak Effect: Usually 1–3 wk.
Duration: 45 days.

Interaction/Toxicity: Amiodarone increases serum levels of digoxin, potentiates warfarin anticoagulants, and may cause bradycardia or sinus arrest in patients receiving β-blockers, calcium antagonists, or lidocaine.

Guidelines/Precautions

1. Because of risk of sinus arrest in patients receiving halothane, have available temporary artificial cardiac (ventricular) pacemakers and sympathomimetics (β-agonists).
2. Thyroid function may be altered.
3. Contraindicated in severe sinus dysfunction, causing marked sinus bradycardia, second-degree and third-degree atrioventricular (AV) block.
4. Discontinue if blurring of vision occurs.
5. Monitor pulmonary toxicity. Perform periodic chest x-ray, pulmonary function tests, and clinical evaluation q3–6mo.

Principal Adverse Reactions

Cardiovascular: Arrhythmias, CHF.
Pulmonary: Pulmonary inflammation or fibrosis.
CNS: Peripheral neuropathy, tremors, involuntary movements.
GI: Hepatitis, cirrhosis.
Eyes: Corneal deposits.
Metabolic: Hyperthyroidism, hypothyroidism.
Dermatologic: Photosensitivity.

AMRINONE LACTATE (INOCOR)

Use(s): Inotropic agent, short-term management of CHF.
Dosing: Loading, IV: 0.75 mg/kg.
     Infusion: 2–20 µg/kg/min.
Elimination: Renal, hepatic.
How Supplied: Injection, 5 mg/mL.

Dilution for Infusion: 500 mg in 500 mL NS solution (1 mg/mL).

Pharmacology

Amrinone inhibits phosphodiesterase and increases intracellular cyclic AMP, which potentiates delivery of calcium ions to the myocardial contractile system. This produces a dose-dependent positive inotropic effect. Peripheral vasodilation is caused by direct vascular smooth muscle relaxation.

Pharmacokinetics

Onset of Action: Within 5 min.
Peak Effect: 10 min.
Duration of Action: 30 min–2 hr.
Interaction/Toxicity: Excessive hypotension with concomitant use of disopyramide; chemical reaction with dextrose containing solutions; thrombocytopenia, hepatic dysfunction with chronic therapy; potentiates inotropic, chronotropic, and arrhythmogenic response to catecholamines and theophylline.

Guidelines/Precautions

1. Use with caution in hypotensive patients.
2. Avoid exposure of ampule to light.
3. Do not mix in solutions containing dextrose or furosemide.
4. Contains metabisulfite. Contraindicated in patients hypersensitive to bisulfites.
5. May aggravate outflow tract obstruction in patients with aortic or pulmonary valvular disease or obstructive cardiomyopathy.

Principal Adverse Reactions

Cardiovascular: Arrhythmia, hypotension.
Hematologic: Thrombocytopenia.
GI: Abdominal pain, hepatic dysfunction.
Other: Hypersensitivity reactions.

ATENOLOL (TENORMIN)

Use(s): Antihypertensive; antianginal; treatment of acute myocardial infarction, acute alcohol withdrawal; migraine prophylaxis.

Dosing: Hypertension/angina: PO, 50–200 mg once daily.
Acute myocardial infarction: IV, 5 mg over 5 min, and IV, 5 mg 10 min later, then PO, 100 mg once daily or 50 mg bid. Dilute IV dose in D_5W or NS solution.
Alcohol withdrawal/migraine prophylaxis: PO, 50–100 mg once daily.

Elimination: Renal.

How Supplied: Tablets: 50 mg, 100 mg.
Injection: 5 mg/10 mL.

Pharmacology

Atenolol is a cardioselective β-blocking agent without membrane stabilizing or intrinsic sympathomimetic (agonist) activities. The cardioselectivity is relative, and in high doses the drug blocks both β_1- and β_2-receptors. It decreases myocardial contractility, heart rate, and blood pressure, which leads to a reduction in myocardial oxygen requirements.

Pharmacokinetics

Onset of Action: PO, <1 hr.
Peak Effect: PO, 2–4 hr.
Duration: PO, 24 hr.
Interaction/Toxicity: The hypotensive effects of atenolol are potentiated by volatile anesthetics, catecholamine-depleting drugs (e.g., reserpine), and calcium channel blockers. Atenolol may unmask negative inotropic effects of ketamine, prolong the elevation of plasma potassium after the administration of succinylcholine, and mask the tachycardia associated with hypoglycemia.

Guidelines/Precautions

1. The drug should be discontinued slowly, especially in patients subject to myocardial ischemia.
2. Use with caution in asthma, heart failure, and AV block greater than first degree.
3. More water soluble and more dependent on renal clearance mechanisms than most other β-blockers.
4. Manifestations of excessive vagal tone and myocardial depression (profound bradycardia, hypotension) may be corrected with IV atropine (1–2 mg), IV isoproterenol (0.02–0.15 µg/kg/min), IV glucagon (1–5 mg), or a transvenous cardiac pacemaker.

Principal Adverse Reactions

Cardiovascular: Hypotension, bradyarrhythmias, rebound angina.
Pulmonary: Bronchospasm, dyspnea, cough.
CNS: Fatigue, depression, disorientation.
GI: Nausea, vomiting, pancreatitis.
Hematologic: Thrombocytopenic purpura.
Musculoskeletal: Arthralgia.

ATRACURIUM BESYLATE (TRACRIUM)

Use(s): Nondepolarizing muscle relaxant.
Dosing: Paralyzing: IV, 0.3–0.5 mg/kg.
  Pretreatment/maintenance: IV, 0.1–0.2 mg/kg.
  Infusion: 2–15 μg/kg/min.
Elimination: Plasma (Hoffman elimination, ester hydrolysis), hepatic, renal.
How Supplied: Injection, 10 mg/mL.
Dilution for Infusion: 20 mg in 100 mL D_5W or NS solution (0.2 mg/mL); 50 mg in 100 mL D_5W or NS solution (0.5 mg/mL).

Pharmacology

Atracurium is a short-acting nondepolarizing skeletal muscle relaxant. It competes for cholinergic receptors at the motor end plate. The duration of neuromuscular blockade is one third that of pancuronium at equipotent doses. It undergoes rapid metabolism via Hoffman elimination and nonspecific enzymatic ester hydrolysis. The primary metabolite is laudanosine, a cerebral stimulant excreted primarily in the urine. Repeated doses or continuous infusion have less cumulative effect on recovery rate than other muscle relaxants. Histamine release and hemodynamic changes are minimal within the recommended dose range and when administered slowly. Higher doses (> 0.5 mg/kg) may lead to moderate histamine release, decreased arterial pressure, and increased heart rate.

Pharmacokinetics

Onset of Action: <3 min.
Peak Effect: 3–5 min.
Duration: 20–35 min.

Interaction/Toxicity: Effects potentiated by prior administration of succinylcholine, volatile anesthetics, aminoglycoside antibiotics, small doses of local anesthetics, loop diuretics, magnesium, lithium, ganglionic blocking drugs, hypothermia, hypokalemia, and respiratory acidosis; enhanced neuromuscular blockade will occur in patients with myasthenia gravis or inadequate adrenocortical function; effects antagonized by anticholinesterase inhibitors, such as neostigmine, edrophonium, and pyridostigmine; increased resistance or reversal of effects with use of theophylline and in patients with burn injury and paresis.

Guidelines/Precautions

1. Monitor response with peripheral nerve stimulator to minimize risk of overdosage.
2. Use with caution in patients with history of bronchial asthma and anaphylactoid reactions.
3. Reverse effects with anticholinesterases such as pyridostigmine bromide, neostigmine, or edrophonium in conjunction with atropine or glycopyrrolate.
4. Pretreatment doses may induce a degree of neuromuscular blockade sufficient to cause hypoventilation in some patients.

Principal Adverse Reactions

Cardiovascular: Hypotension, vasodilation, sinus tachycardia, sinus bradycardia.
Pulmonary: Hypoventilation, apnea, bronchospasm, laryngospasm, dyspnea.
Musculoskeletal: Inadequate block, prolonged block.
Dermatologic: Rash, urticaria.

ATROPINE SULFATE (ATROPINE SULFATE)

Use(s): Cholinergic antagonist.
Dosing: Premedication and vagolysis IV/IM: Adults: 0.4–1.0 mg. Children: 10–20 µg/kg (minimum dose, 0.1 mg). PO, 30 µg/kg. Use higher potency injectate solutions (>0.3 mg/mL) and dilute in 3–5 mL apple juice or carbonated cola beverage.

Reversal of neuromuscular blockade: 0.015 mg/kg IV
   with anticholinesterase neostigmine (0.05 mg/kg IV)
   or edrophonium (0.5–1 mg/kg IV).
Bronchodilation Inhalation: Adults: 0.025 mg/kg q4–
   6h. Children: 0.05 mg/kg q4–6h. Maximum dose
   2.5 mg. Dilute to 2–3 mL with NS solution and deliver by compressed air nebulizer.

Elimination: Hepatic, renal.
How Supplied: Injection: 0.05 mg/mL, 0.1 mg/mL, 0.3 mg/
mL, 0.4 mg/mL, 0.5 mg/mL, 0.8 mg/mL, 1 mg/mL. Inhalation
solution: 0.2%, 0.5%; tablets: 0.4 mg, 0.6 mg.

Pharmacology

Atropine competitively antagonizes the action of acetylcholine at
the muscarinic receptor. It decreases salivary, bronchial, and gastric secretions and relaxes bronchial smooth muscle. Gastrointestinal tone and motility are reduced. Lower esophageal sphincter
pressure decreases, and intraocular pressure increases (because of
pupillary dilation). Large doses may increase body temperature by
preventing sweat secretion. Peripheral vagal blockade of the sinus
and AV node increases heart rate. Transient decreases in heart
rate by small doses reflects the CNS effect of the drug. Atropine
is a tertiary amine and therefore crosses the blood-brain barrier. In
high doses it stimulates and then depresses the medullary and
higher cerebral centers.

Pharmacokinetics

Onset of Action: IV, almost immediate; inhalation, 3–5 min.
Peak Effect: IV, 2 min; inhalation, 1–2 hr.
Duration of Action: IV/IM, 1–2 hr; inhalation, 3–6 hr.
Interaction/Toxicity: Additive anticholinergic effects with antihistamines, phenothiazines, tricyclic antidepressants, procainamide, quinidine, MAO inhibitors, benzodiazepines, antipsychot-
ics; increase in intraocular pressure enhanced by nitrates, nitrites,
alkalinizing agents, disopyramide, corticosteroids, haloperidol;
potentiates sympathomimetics; antagonizes anticholinesterases
and metoclopramide; may produce central anticholinergic syndrome (hallucinations, delirium, coma).

Guidelines/Precautions

1. Use with caution in patients with tachyarrhythmias, CHF, acute myocardial ischemia or infarction, fever, esophageal reflux, GI infections.
2. Contraindicated in patients with narrow-angle glaucoma, obstructive uropathy, obstructive disease of the GI tract.
3. May accumulate and produce systemic side effects with multiple dosing by inhalation, especially in the elderly.
4. Treat toxicity with sedation (benzodiazepines) and administration of physostigmine.
5. Infants, small children, and elderly patients are more susceptible to systemic effects of atropine, e.g., rapid and irregular pulse, fever, excitement, agitation.

Principal Adverse Reactions

Cardiovascular: Tachycardia (high doses), bradycardia (low doses), palpitations.
Pulmonary: Respiratory depression.
CNS: Confusion, hallucinations, nervousness.
GU: Urinary hesitancy, retention.
GI: Gastroesophageal reflux.
Eyes: Mydriasis, blurred vision, increased intraocular pressure.
Dermatologic: Urticaria.
Other: Decreased sweating, allergic reaction.

BENZOCAINE (AMERICAINE, HURRICAINE, DERMOPLAST, RHULICAINE, SOLARCAINE)

Use(s): Topical anesthesia.
Dosing: Topical.
Elimination: Plasma cholinesterase.
How Supplied: Aerosol, cream, ointment 0.5%–20%.

Pharmacology

An ester of benzoic acid with a rapid onset of action and short duration. It stabilizes neuronal membranes by inhibiting ionic fluxes required for the initiation and conduction of impulses. There is virtually no systemic absorption.

Pharmacokinetics

Onset of Action: 15–30 sec.
Peak Effect: 1 min.
Duration of Action: 12–15 min.
Interaction/Toxicity: Metabolite (*p*-aminobenzoic acid [PABA]) inhibits action of sulfonamides.

Guidelines/Precautions

1. Do not use in the eyes or areas with secondary bacterial infection.
2. Not for injection.
3. Not for prolonged use.

Principal Adverse Reactions

Cardiovascular: Hypotension.
Pulmonary: Respiratory depression.
CNS: Seizures.
Dermatologic: Urticaria, pruritus, anaphylactoid reactions (rare).
Other: Methemoglobinemia.

BRETYLIUM TOSYLATE (BRETYLOL)

Use(s): Class III antiarrhythmic for ventricular fibrillation and arrhythmias.
Dosing: IV loading/IM: ventricular tachycardia: 5–10 mg/kg over 15 min; may be repeated in 1–2 hr
IV loading: ventricular fibrillation: 5–10 mg/kg over 1 min (q15–30 min to maximum 30 mg/kg).
Infusion: 1–2 mg/min.
Therapeutic level: 0.5–1.0 μg/mL.
Elimination: Renal.
How Supplied: Injection: 50 mg/mL.
Dilution for Infusion: 2 g in 500 ml D_5W or NS solution (4 mg/mL).

Pharmacology

Bretylium initially releases norepinephrine from sympathetic ganglia and postganglionic adrenergic neurons. This initial action may account for increased heart rate, irritability, and blood pressure. Subsequently there is inhibition of release of norepinephrine in response to sympathetic nerve stimulation. The adrenergic blockade depends on uptake of bretylium by adrenergic neurons and may lead to orthostatic hypotension and bradycardia. Cardiac performance is not significantly changed, but pulmonary artery pressure may be increased. Bretylium increases ventricular fibrillation threshold and suppresses ventricular arrhythmias. The electrophysiological effects include an increase in action potential duration and effective refractory period, an increase in ventricular conduction velocity and a decrease in the disparity between normal and damaged cells.

Pharmacokinetics

Onset of Action: IV: antifibrillatory: few minutes; IV/IM: suppression of ventricular arrhythmia: 20 min–2 hr.
Peak Effect: IV: antifibrillatory: 20 min–2 hr; IV/IM: suppression of ventricular arrhythmia: 6–9 hr.
Duration of Action: IV/IM: 6–24 hr.
Interaction/Toxicity: Initial release of norepinephrine may worsen arrhythmias caused by cardiac glycoside toxicity; resistance to anti-adrenergic effects in patients receiving tricyclic antidepressants, which block the uptake of bretylium.

Guidelines/Precautions

1. Use with caution in patients with pheochromocytoma, aortic stenosis, and pulmonary hypertension.
2. Treat severe hypotension with appropriate fluid therapy and vasopressor agents such as dopamine or norepinephrine.

Principal Adverse Reactions

Cardiovascular: Hypotension, transitory hypertension and arrhythmias, anginal attacks.
Pulmonary: Shortness of breath.
CNS: Dizziness, syncope.
GI: Nausea, vomiting, diarrhea, abdominal pain.
Other: Rash, hiccups.

BUPIVACAINE HCL (MARCAINE, SENSORCAINE)

Use(s): Regional anesthesia.
Dosing: Infiltration/peripheral nerve block: <150 mg (0.25%–0.5% solution).

IV regional: Upper extremities: 100–125 mg (40–50 mL of 0.25% solution).

Lower extremities: 125–150 mg (100–120 mL of 0.125% solution). Do not add epinephrine for IV regional block.

Brachial plexus block: 75–150 mg (30–40 mL of 0.25%–0.375% solution). Children, 0.2–0.33 mL/kg.

Caudal: 37.5–150 mg (15–30 mL of 0.25% or 0.5% solution). Children: 0.4–0.7 mL/kg (L2–T10 level of anesthesia).

Epidural: Bolus, 50–150 mg (0.25%–0.75% solution). Children, 1.5–2.5 mg/kg (0.25%–0.5% solution). Infusion, 8–12 ml/hr (0.125%) solution. Children, 0.2–0.35 mL/kg/hr.

Rate of onset and potency of local anesthetic action may be enhanced by carbonation. (Add 0.1 mL of 8.4% sodium bicarbonate with 20 mL of 0.25%–0.5% bupivacaine. Do not use if there is precipitation.)

Spinal: Bolus/infusion, 7–15 mg (0.75% solution). Children: 0.5 mg/kg, with a minimum of 1 mg. Add 10–20 μg of epinephrine if desired.

Intrapleural: Bolus, 20 mL (0.4 ml/kg [0.5% solution; add epinephrine 1:200,000 if desired]). Infusion, 5–7 mL/hr (0.125 mL/kg/hr [0.25% solution]).

Maximum safe dose: 2 mg/kg without epinephrine. 2–3 mg/kg with epinephrine.

Solutions containing preservatives should not be used for epidural or caudal block.

Elimination: Hepatic, pulmonary.

How Supplied: Injection: 0.25%, 0.5%, 0.75% with and without epinephrine 1:200,000.

Dilution for Infusion: Epidural use only. 20 mL 0.25% in 20 mL (preservative-free) NS (0.125%) solution.

Pharmacology

This amino amide local anesthetic stabilizes neuronal membranes by inhibiting ionic fluxes required for the initiation and conduction of impulses. The progression of anesthesia is related to the diameter, myelination, and conduction velocity of affected nerve fibers with order of loss of function being (1) autonomic, (2) pain,

(3) temperature, (4) touch, (5) proprioception, and (6) skeletal muscle tone. The onset of action is reasonably rapid, and duration is significantly longer than with any other commonly used local anesthetic. Addition of epinephrine only marginally increases duration of effect. Hypotension results from loss of sympathetic tone, as in spinal or epidural anesthesia. Compared with other amides, there is more cardiotoxicity with intravascular injection.

Pharmacokinetics

Onset of Action: Infiltration, 2–10 min; epidural, 4–17 min; spinal, <1 min.

Peak Effect: Infiltration and epidural, 30–45 min; spinal, 15 min.

Duration of Action: Infiltration/epidural/spinal, 200–400 min (prolonged with epinephrine); intrapleural, 48 hr.

Interaction/Toxicity: Prior use of chloroprocaine may interfere with action; seizures, respiratory and circulatory depression at high plasma levels; reduced clearance with concomitant use of β-blocking agents, cimetidine; benzodiazepines increase seizure threshold, duration of local or regional anesthesia prolonged by vasoconstrictor agents, e.g., epinephrine; reduced dose requirements in pregnant patients.

Guidelines/Precautions

1. Not recommended for obstetrical paracervical block (may cause fetal bradycardia, death).
2. Concentrations above 0.5% are not recommended for use in obstetrics due to incidence of intractable cardiac arrest. The increased cardiac toxicity of bupivacaine (compared with lidocaine or mepivacaine) results from a greater decrease in myocardial contractility and depression of cardiac conduction.
3. Cauda equina syndrome with permanent neurologic deficit may occur in patients receiving >15 mg of a 0.75% bupivacaine solution with a continuous spinal technique.
4. IV access is essential during major regional block.
5. Use with caution in patients with hypovolemia, severe CHF, shock, and all forms of heart block.
6. In IV regional blocks, deflate the cuff after 40 min and not <20 min. Between 20 and 40 min, the cuff can be deflated,

reinflated immediately, and finally deflated after 1 min to reduce the sudden absorption of anesthetic into the systemic circulation.
7. Contraindicated in patients with hypersensitivity to amide type local anesthetics.
8. Toxic plasma levels of bupivacaine (all local anesthetics), e.g., from accidental intravascular injection, may cause cardiopulmonary collapse and seizures. Premonitory signs and symptoms are numbness of the tongue and circumoral tissues, metallic taste, restlessness, tinnitus, and tremors. Support of circulation (IV fluids, vasopressors, defibrillation) and securing a patent airway (ventilate with 100% oxygen) are paramount. Thiopental (1–2 mg/kg IV), midazolam (0.02–0.04 mg/kg IV), or diazepam (0.1 mg/kg IV) may be used for prophylaxis and/or treatment of seizures.
9. The level of sympathetic blockade (bradycardia with block above T5) determines the degree of hypotension (often heralded by nausea vomiting) following epidural or intrathecal bupivacaine (or other local anesthetic). Fluid hydration (10–20 mL/kg NS or lactated Ringer's solution), vasopressor agents, e.g., ephedrine and left uterine displacement in pregnant patients, may be used for prophylaxis and/or treatment. Administer atropine to treat bradycardia.
10. Epidural, caudal, or intrathecal injections should be avoided when the patient has hypovolemic shock, septicemia, infection at the injection site, or coagulopathy.

Principal Adverse Reactions

Cardiovascular: Hypotension, arrhythmias, cardiac arrest.
Pulmonary: Respiratory impairment, arrest.
CNS: Seizures, tinnitus, blurred vision.
Allergic: Urticaria, angioneurotic edema, anaphylactoid symptoms.
Epidural/Caudal/Spinal: High spinal, hypotension, urinary retention, lower extremity weakness and paralysis, loss of sphincter control, headache, backache, cranial nerve palsies, slowing of labor.

BUTORPHANOL TARTRATE (STADOL)*

Use(s): Analgesia.
Dosing: IM: 1–4 mg q3–4h.
          IV: 0.5–2 mg q3–4h.
          Epidural bolus: 1–2 mg. Dilute in 10 mL local anes-
          thetic or (preservative-free) NS solution.
Elimination: Hepatic, renal.
How Supplied: Injection: 1 mg/mL, 2 mg/mL.

Pharmacology

A synthetic benzomorphan derivative. It is a potent opioid agonist-antagonist (partial agonist) with analgesic potency 3.5–7 times that of morphine or 30–40 times that of meperidine. Butorphanol has a ceiling effect for respiratory depression at 30–60 μg/kg. Analgesic doses increase systemic blood pressure, pulmonary artery blood pressure, and cardiac output. Analgesia is not adequate for the performance of surgery.

Pharmacokinetics

Onset of Action: IV, 1–5 min; IM, 10 min.
Peak Effect: IV, 5–10 min; IM, 30–60 min.
Duration of Action: IV, 2–4 hr; IM/epidural, 3–4 hr.
Interaction/Toxicity: Decreases effectiveness of opioid agonists; may precipitate withdrawal in opioid-dependent patients; additive effects with phenothiazines, droperidol, barbiturates, and other tranquilizers.

Guidelines/Precautions

1. Slight increase in systolic blood pressure when used for premedication.
2. May cause respiratory depression.
3. Use with caution in patients who have been chronically receiving opiate agonists. High doses may precipitate withdrawal symptoms as a result of opiate antagonist effect.
4. Crosses the placental barrier; usage in labor may produce depression of respiration in the neonate. Resuscitation may be required; have naloxone available.
5. Drug increases cardiac work and should be used with caution in patients with ischemic disease.

*For epidural/intrathecal precautions, see Alfentanil, Guidelines/Precautions, items 5 and 6, pp 4–5.

Principal Adverse Reactions

Cardiovascular: Hypertension, hypotension, palpitations.
Pulmonary: Respiratory depression.
CNS: Euphoria, hallucinations, sedation, headache.
GI: Nausea, vomiting.
Autonomic: Flushing, dry mouth, sensitivity to cold.

CALCIUM CHLORIDE (CALCIUM CHLORIDE)

Use(s): Electrolyte replacement, positive inotrope, treatment of hyperkalemia, hypermagnesemia, and calcium antagonist overdose.
Dosing: IV, 500–1000 mg (10 mg/kg), 2%–10% solution. Do not exceed rate of 1 mL/min. Maintain serum calcium levels at 8.5–10 mg/dL.
Elimination: GI, renal.
How Supplied: Injection: 10% solution.

Pharmacology

Calcium is essential for maintenance of the functional integrity of nervous, muscular, and skeletal systems, cell membrane and capillary permeability. It is also essential for contraction of cardiac, smooth and skeletal muscles, renal function, respiration, and blood coagulation. Increase in cardiac output follows an increase in myocardial contractility and a decrease in peripheral vascular resistance and is associated with a decreased heart rate. 10% calcium chloride is more irritating to the veins and provides 3 times more calcium (270 mg/13.5 mEq/g) than an equal volume of 10% calcium gluconate (90 mg/4.5 mEq/g).

Pharmacokinetics

Onset of Action: <30 sec (electrolyte replacement and inotropic effects).
Peak Effect: <1 min (electrolyte replacement and inotropic effects).
Duration of Action: 10–20 min (inotropic effects).
Interaction/Toxicity: May precipitate arrhythmias in digitalized patients; antagonizes effects of verapamil and other calcium chan-

nel blockers, magnesium; sloughing and necrosis with extravasation, IM or SC injection; complexes with tetracycline antibiotics when mixed; chemically incompatible in parenteral admixtures of carbonates, phosphates, sulfates, or tartrates.

Guidelines/Precautions

1. IV injection should be given slowly and through a large vein to minimize venous irritation.
2. Treat extravasation by discontinuing calcium and local infiltration with 1% procaine HCl and hyaluronidase.
3. Hypercalcemia is more dangerous than hypocalcemia. Electrocardiogram (ECG) monitoring and frequent determinations of serum calcium concentrations should be done.
4. Rapid IV injection may cause arrhythmias, hypotension, or hypertension.
5. Inadvertent systemic overloading with calcium ions can produce an acute hypercalcemic syndrome characterized by a markedly elevated plasma calcium level, weakness, lethargy, intractable nausea and vomiting, coma, and sudden death. Treat by immediate discontinuation of calcium, administration of NS infusions ($\leq$6 L/24 hr) and IV furosemide (20–40 mg q2–4 hr). Fluid therapy can be monitored with a central venous pressure (CVP) catheter.
6. Chloride salt is acidifying and should not be used when acidosis coincides with hypocalcemia.
7. Hypocalcemia may develop after rapid transfusion of citrated blood (>2 mL/kg/min) or large volumes of colloid solution. Administer IV calcium, 1.35 mEq/27 mg (adults) or 0.45 mEq/9 mg (children), after every 100 mL of citrated blood.

Principal Adverse Reactions

Cardiovascular: Hypertension, hypotension, bradycardia, arrhythmias, cardiac arrest.
CNS: Lethargy, coma.
Dermatologic: Sloughing, necrosis, abscess formation.
Metabolic: Hypercalcemia.

CALCIUM GLUCONATE (CALCIUM GLUCONATE)

Use(s): Electrolyte replacement, positive inotrope, treatment of hyperkalemia (with ECG changes), hypermagnesemia, and calcium antagonist overdose.

Dosing: IV, 500–2000 mg (30 mg/kg [10% solution]) (do not exceed rate of 1 mL/min).

PO, 500–2000 mg as required;   maintain serum calcium levels at 8.5–10 mg/dL.

Elimination: GI, renal.

How Supplied: Injection: 10% solution; tablets: 500 mg (45 mg calcium), 650 mg (58.5 mg calcium), 1 g (90 mg calcium).

Pharmacology

Calcium is essential for maintenance of the functional integrity of nervous, muscular, and skeletal systems, cell membrane, and capillary permeability. It is also essential for contraction of cardiac, smooth, and skeletal muscles, renal function, respiration, and blood coagulation. Increase in cardiac output follows an increase in myocardial contractility; a decrease in peripheral vascular resistance is associated with a decreased heart rate. 10% calcium gluconate is less irritating to the veins and provides 3 times less calcium (90 mg/4.5 mEq/g) than an equal volume of 10% calcium chloride (270 mg/13.5 mEq/g).

Pharmacokinetics

Onset of Action: IV, <30 sec (electrolyte replacement and inotropic effects).

Peak Effect: IV, <1 min (electrolyte replacement and inotropic effects).

Duration of Action: IV, 10–20 min (inotropic effects).

Interaction/Toxicity: May precipitate arrhythmias in digitalized patients; antagonizes effects of verapamil and other calcium channel blockers, magnesium; sloughing and necrosis with extravasation, IM or SC injection; complexes with tetracycline antibiotics when mixed; chemically incompatible in parenteral admixtures of carbonates, phosphates, sulfates, or tartrates; rapid IV injection may cause peripheral vasodilation and hypotension.

Guidelines/Precautions

1. IV injection should be done slowly and through a large vein to minimize venous irritation.
2. Treat extravasation by discontinuing calcium and local infiltration with 1% procaine HCl and hyaluronidase.
3. Hypercalcemia is more dangerous than hypocalcemia. ECG monitoring and frequent determinations of serum calcium concentrations should be done.
4. Rapid IV injection may cause arrhythmias, hypotension, or hypertension.
5. Inadvertent systemic overloading with calcium ions can produce an acute hypercalcemic syndrome characterized by a markedly elevated plasma calcium level, weakness, lethargy, intractable nausea and vomiting, coma, and sudden death. Treat by immediate discontinuation of calcium, administration of NS infusions (≤6 L/24 hr) and IV furosemide (20–40 mg q2–4h). Fluid therapy can be monitored with a CVP catheter.
6. Hypocalcemia may develop after rapid transfusion of citrated blood (>2 mL/kg/min) or large volumes of colloid solution. Administer IV calcium, 1.35 mEq/27 mg (adults) or 0.45 mEq/9 mg (children), after every 100 mL of citrated blood.

Principal Adverse Reactions

Cardiovascular: Hypertension, hypotension, bradycardia, arrhythmias, cardiac arrest.
CNS: Lethargy, coma.
Dermatologic: Sloughing, necrosis, abscess formation.
Metabolic: Hypercalcemia.

CAPTOPRIL (CAPOTEN)

Use(s): Antihypertensive; treatment of CHF, post-MI Ventricular modeling.
Dosing: Hypertension: PO, 12.5–50 mg bid or tid.
　　　　CHF: PO, 25–100 mg tid to maximum of 450 mg/day.
Elimination: Renal, hepatic.
How Supplied: Tablets: 12.5 mg, 25 mg, 37.5 mg, 50 mg, 100 mg.

Pharmacology

Captopril inhibits angiotensin-converting enzyme (ACE), thereby blocking the conversion of angiotensin I to angiotensin II. Angiotensin II is a potent vasoconstrictor and acts to release aldosterone. Thus, captopril lowers total peripheral vascular resistance and blood pressure and inhibits water and salt retention normally produced by aldosterone. It lowers both preload and afterload. ACE is also responsible for the metabolism of bradykinin, a potent vasodilatory autacoid. Bradykinin levels in tissue increase after captopril.

Pharmacokinetics

Onset of Action: 15 min.
Peak Effect: 60–90 min.
Duration of Action: 2–6 hr.
Interaction/Toxicity: Additive hypotensive effects with diuretics, vasodilators, β-blockers, calcium channel blockers, volatile anesthetics; elevates serum potassium levels, which may be significant with renal insufficiency and use of potassium-sparing diuretics such as spironolactone, triamterene, or amiloride; antihypertensive effect antagonized by indomethacin and other nonsteroidal anti-inflammatory drugs.

Guidelines/Precautions

1. May be associated with angioedema, bone marrow suppression, and proteinuria. Emergency therapy for angioedema with airway obstruction should include SC epinephrine 1:1000 (0.5–1.0 mg).
2. May cause profound first-dose hypotension, particularly in those patients who are volume depleted or when used concomitantly with agents that reduce vascular volume. Treat hypotension with volume expansion.
3. Should not be used with potassium-sparing diuretics because of the possibility of hyperkalemia.
4. May be associated with a persistent, dry cough resistant to normal antitussives, but which may respond to a decrease in dose.
5. Use with caution in hypertensive patients with renal disease. Increases in blood urea nitrogen (BUN) and serum creatinine levels may develop after reduction of blood pressure. Monitor renal function during the first few weeks of therapy.

6. In patients with CHF, treatment with captopril may be associated with oliguria or progressive azotemia and, rarely, with acute renal failure or death.
7. Use in pregnancy associated with increased cranial facial dysplasias, other fetal abnormalities.

Principal Adverse Reactions

Cardiovascular: Hypotension, palpitations, tachycardia.
Pulmonary: Cough, dyspnea.
CNS: Dizziness, fatigue.
GI: Abdominal pain, dysgeusia, peptic ulcer.
Dermatologic: Rash, pruritus.
Renal: Elevation of BUN and creatinine levels, proteinuria, renal failure.
Hematologic: Neutropenia, thrombocytopenia, hemolytic anemia, eosinophilia.
Other: Angioedema, lymphadenopathy.

CHLORDIAZEPOXIDE HCL (LIBRIUM)

Use(s): Premedication, sedative/hypnotic, treatment of acute alcohol withdrawal.
Dosing: Premedication: PO, 5–10 mg (0.2 mg/kg); IM, 50–100 mg (1–2 mg/kg).
  Withdrawal symptoms: IM, IV, and PO, 50–100 mg (dilute in 5 mL NS solution or sterile water). Repeat in 2–4 hr if necessary. Do not use IM diluent for IV administration.
Elimination: Hepatic.
How Supplied: Injection, 5 mL dry, filled ampule containing 100 mg chlordiazepoxide and a 2-mL ampule of special IM diluent; tablets, 5 mg, 10 mg, 25 mg.

Pharmacology

This benzodiazepine increases γ-aminobutyric acid (GABA) neurotransmission in the CNS. The drug exerts antianxiety, sedative, appetite-stimulating, and weak analgesic effects. Chlordiazepoxide may possess some peripheral anticholinergic activity. It has minimal depressant effects on ventilation and circulation in the absence of other CNS depressant drugs. Prolonged recovery.

Pharmacokinetics

Onset: IV, few minutes; IM/PO, 15–30 min.
Peak Effect: IV, 5 min; IM/PO, 45 min.
Duration: IV, 15 min–1 hr; IM/PO, 2–6 hr.
Interaction/Toxicity: Potentiates sedative CNS and circulatory depressant effect of narcotics, alcohol, sedative-hypnotics, phenothiazines, MAO inhibitors; reduces requirements for volatile anesthetics; elimination decreased by cimetidine, propranolol; effects antagonized by flumazenil.

Guidelines/Precautions

1. Reduce dosage in elderly, hypovolemic, or high-risk surgical patients, and with concomitant use of narcotics and other sedatives.
2. Paradoxical reactions (excitement, stimulation) in hyperactive aggressive children and psychiatric patients.
3. Treat overdosage with supportive measures and flumazenil. (slow IV, 0.2–1 mg).

Principal Adverse Reactions

Cardiovascular: Hypotension, tachycardia.
Pulmonary: Hypoventilation, apnea.
CNS: Drowsiness, ataxia, confusion.
Hematologic: Agranulocytosis.
Other: Hepatic dysfunction.

CHLOROPROCAINE HCL (NESACAINE)*

Use(s): Regional anesthesia.
Dosing: Infiltration and peripheral nerve block: <40 mL (1%–2% solution).

Epidural: Bolus, 10–25 mL (2%–3% solution) (approximately 1.5–2 mL for each segment to be anesthetized) (repeat doses at 40- to 60-min intervals); infusion, 30 mL/hr (0.5% solution).

*For additional precautions, see Bupivacaine, Guidelines/Precautions, items 8 to 10, p. 20.

Caudal: 10–25 mL (2% to 3% solution). Children: 0.4–0.7 mL/kg (L2–T10 level of anesthesia). Repeat doses at 40- to 60-min intervals.

Rate of onset and potency of local anesthetic action may be enhanced by carbonation. (Add 1 mL of 8.4% sodium bicarbonate with 30 mL of 2%–3% chloroprocaine. Do not use if there is precipitation.) Use preservative-free solution only for epidural or caudal anesthesia.

Maximum safe dose: 800 mg (without epinephrine). 1000 mg (with epinephrine).

Elimination: Plasma cholinesterase.

How Supplied: 1%, 2% preservative-containing solution. 2%, 3% preservative-free solution.

Dilution for Infusion: Epidural use only. 12.5 mL (2%) in 37.5 mL (preservative-free) NS (0.5%) solution.

Pharmacology

A benzoic acid ester and short-acting local anesthetic. It stabilizes the neuronal membrane and prevents the initiation and transmission of impulses. It is rapidly hydrolyzed by plasma pseudocholinesterase. Epinephrine prolongs the duration of action by reducing the rate of absorption and plasma concentration. Decreased myocardial contractility and peripheral vasodilation with toxic blood concentrations, resulting in decreased arterial pressure and cardiac output. Ineffective for topical anesthesia. Chloroprocaine is not recommended for IV regional anesthesia because of the high incidence of thrombophlebitis.

Pharmacokinetics

Onset of Action: Infiltration/epidural, 6–12 min.

Peak Effect: Infiltration/epidural, 10–20 min.

Duration of Action: Infiltration/epidural, 30–60 min (prolonged with epinephrine).

Interaction/Toxicity: Prolongs the effect of succinylcholine; metabolite (PABA) inhibits the action of sulfonamides; toxicity enhanced by cimetidine, anticholinesterases (which inhibits degradation); high plasma levels associated with seizures, respiratory and circulatory depression; duration of local of regional anesthesia prolonged by vasoconstrictor agents, e.g., epinephrine; decreased effectiveness of epidural narcotics with epidural chloroprocaine.

Guidelines/Precautions

1. Do not use for spinal anesthesia.
2. Use with caution in patients with severe disturbances of cardiac rhythm, shock, or heart block.
3. Reduce doses in obstetric, elderly, hypovolemic, high-risk patients and those with increased intra-abdominal pressure.
4. Potential for allergic reaction with repeated use.
5. Contraindicated in patients with hypersensitivity to chloroprocaine or ester-type local anesthetics.
6. Persistent neurologic damage has been noted after accidental spinal anesthesia with large doses of sodium bisulfite containing chloroprocaine solutions.

Principal Adverse Reactions

Cardiovascular: Hypotension, arrhythmias, bradycardia.
Pulmonary: Respiratory depression, arrest.
CNS: Seizures, tinnitus, tremors.
Allergic: Urticaria, pruritus, angioneurotic edema.
Epidural/Caudal/Spinal: High spinal, arachnoiditis, backache, loss of perineal sensation and sexual function, permanent motor, sensory and/or autonomic (sphincter control) deficit of lower segments, slowing of labor.

CHLORPROMAZINE HCL (THORAZINE)

Use(s): Antipsychotic, premedication, antiemetic, and relief of hiccups.
Dosing: Premedication: PO, 25–50 mg (0.5–1 mg/kg); IM, 12.5–25 mg (0.25–0.5 mg/kg).
       Emesis and hiccups: PO/IM, 10–50 mg (0.25–0.55 mg/kg) bid or qid (maximum dosage for children: 40 mg/day <5 yr old, 75 mg/day 5–12 yr old); rectal, 50–100 mg (1.1 mg/kg); IV, 25–50 mg (0.25–0.55 mg/kg). Dilute to 1 mg/mL with NS solution. Give at rate of 1 mg/min. Observe for hypotension with parenteral administration.
Elimination: Hepatic.
How Supplied: Tablets: 10 mg, 25 mg, 50 mg, 100 mg, 200 mg; oral solution: 2 mg/mL; oral concentrate: 30 mg/mL, 100 mg/mL; suppositories: 25 and 100 mg; injection: 25 mg/mL.

Pharmacology

Chlorpromazine is a phenothiazine tranquilizer with antiemetic, antiadrenergic, anticholinergic, and antiserotoninergic actions. The neuroleptic actions are most likely caused by antagonism of dopamine as a synaptic neurotransmitter in the basal ganglia and limbic portions of the forebrain. Extrapyramidal side effects are evidence of interference with the normal actions of dopamine.

Pharmacokinetics

Onset: IV/IM, within 30 min; PO, 30–60 min.
Peak Effect: PO, 2–3 hr.
Duration: PO, 4–6 hr; IM, 3–4 hr.
Interaction/Toxicity: Potentiates barbiturates, narcotics, anesthetics; lithium reduces bioavailability; mephentermine, epinephrine, thiazide diuretics potentiate chlorpromazine-induced hypotension; interferes with metabolism of phenytoin (Dilantin) and may precipitate toxicity; concomitant administration of propranolol increases plasma levels of both drugs.

Guidelines/Precautions

1. May suppress laryngeal reflex with possible aspiration of vomitus.
2. May lower convulsive threshold.
3. Use cautiously in geriatric patients, patients with glaucoma, prostatic hypertrophy, seizure disorders, and children with acute illnesses (e.g., chickenpox, measles).
4. Neuroleptic malignant syndrome, a rare side effect, may be treated symptomatically and with dantrolene.
5. Extrapyramidal reactions may consist of dystonic reactions, feelings of motor restlessness (akathisia), and parkinsonian signs and symptoms. Dystonic reactions occur more frequently in children, especially those with acute infections, whereas parkinsonian symptoms predominate in geriatric patients. Therapy should include discontinuation of chlorpromazine, or reduction in dosage, and treatment with an anticholinergic antiparkinsonian agent (e.g., benztropine, trihexyphenidyl) or with diphenhydramine (IV/PO, 25 mg). Maintenance of an adequate airway should be instituted if necessary.

6. Do not use epinephrine to treat chlorpromazine-induced hypotension. Phenothiazines cause a reversal of epinephrine's vasopressor effects and a further lowering of blood pressure. Treat the drug-induced hypotension with norepinephrine or phenylephrine.

Principal Adverse Reactions

Cardiovascular: Hypotension, tachycardia.
CNS: Extrapyramidal reactions, seizures, drowsiness.
Allergic: Urticaria, photosensitivity.
Hematologic: Agranulocytosis, hemolytic anemia.
Other: Neuroleptic malignant syndrome.

CIMETIDINE (TAGAMET)

Use(s): Treatment of peptic ulcer, pathologic hypersecretory states; prophylaxis against acid pulmonary aspiration.
Dosing: PO, 300 mg (7.5 mg/kg) q6–8h (alternately 400–1600 mg at bedtime).
   IV/IM, 300 mg (7.5 mg/kg) q6–8h.
Elimination: Renal, hepatic.
How Supplied: Tablets: 200 mg, 300 mg, 400 mg, 800 mg; oral solution: 60 mg/mL; injection: 150 mg/mL.
Dilution for Infusion: 300 mg in 50 mL D_5W or NS solution (6 mg/mL). Infuse over 15–20 min.

Pharmacology

Cimetidine is a competitive histamine H_2 receptor antagonist that blocks the effects of histamine, pentagastrin, and acetylcholine on gastric acid secretion. It has no significant effect on gastric emptying time, volume, lower esophageal sphincter tone, or pancreatic secretions.

Pharmacokinetics

Onset: PO/IV, <45 min.
Peak Effect: PO/IV, 45–90 min.
Duration: PO, 6–8 hr; IV, 4–4.5 hr.

Interaction/Toxicity: May inhibit metabolism of benzodiazepines, caffeine, calcium-channel blockers, carbamazepine, chloroquine, labetalol, lidocaine, metoprolol, metronidazole, pentoxifylline, phenytoin, propranolol, quinidine, quinine, sulfonylureas, theophyllines, triamterene, tricyclic antidepressants, and coumarin anticoagulants; decreases renal tubular secretion of procainamide; may decrease serum concentrations of digoxin; may decrease effects of tocainide; increases the neuromuscular blocking effects of succinylcholine; absorption of cimetidine may be decreased by antacids, anticholinergics, and metoclopramide.

Guidelines/Precautions

1. Rapid IV administration may produce hypotension, bradycardia, or heart block.
2. Use with caution in elderly patients because it may produce CNS dysfunction (e.g., confusion, agitation, seizures).
3. May increase airway resistance in patients with bronchial asthma, reflecting loss of H_2 receptor–mediated bronchodilation, leaving unopposed H_1 receptor–mediated bronchoconstriction.

Principal Adverse Reactions

Cardiovascular: Bradycardia, arrhythmias.
CNS: Dizziness, somnolence, confusion, disorientation, seizures.
GI: Diarrhea.
Dermatologic: Rash.
Musculoskeletal: Arthralgia.
Endocrine: Gynecomastia.
Hematologic: Agranulocytosis, aplastic anemia, thrombocytopenia.
Renal: Minor reversible elevations of serum creatinine level.

CLONIDINE HCL (CATAPRES)*

Use(s): Antihypertensive, treatment of opioid/alcohol withdrawal states, epidural/spinal analgesia; supplementation of anesthesia.

*For epidural/intrathecal precautions, see Alfentanil, Guidelines/Precautions, item 6, pp. 4–5.

Dosing: PO, 0.1–1.5 mg/day; sublingual, 0.2–0.4 mg/day.
Transdermal, 0.1–0.3 mg once q7d.
Epidural bolus, 150–800 µg (2–10 µg/kg) continuous 10–20 µg/hr.
Spinal bolus, 15–30 µg.

Elimination: Renal, hepatic.

How Supplied: Tablets: 0.1 mg, 0.2 mg, or 0.3 mg; transdermal therapeutic system: releases 0.1, 0.2, 0.3 mg/24 hr; parenteral form: Not currently available for general clinical use in the United States.

Pharmacology

Clonidine inhibits central sympathetic outflow through activation of α_2-adrenergic receptors in the medullary vasomotor center. It decreases blood pressure, heart rate, and cardiac output. Rebound hypertension occurs when therapy is discontinued abruptly. Clonidine suppresses signs and symptoms of opioid withdrawal by replacing opioid-mediated inhibition with α_2-mediated inhibition of CNS sympathetic activity. It acts on opioid receptors of the substantia gelatinosa in the spinal cord. As an anesthetic adjunct, clonidine reduces requirements for opioids and inhalation anesthetics, prolongs regional block, and enhances postoperative analgesia.

Pharmacokinetics

Onset of Action: PO, 30–60 min; epidural/spinal, <15 min; transdermal, <2 days.

Peak Effect: PO, 2–4 hr; transdermal, 2–3 days.

Duration of Action: PO, 8 hr; epidural/spinal, 3–4 hr; transdermal, 7 days.

Interaction/Toxicity: Potentiates effects of opioids, alcohol, barbiturates, sedatives; decreases the requirements for volatile anesthetics; effect reduced with use of tricyclic antidepressant, naloxone; addition of clonidine to epidural or spinal anesthetics or narcotics increases duration of pain relief and may be accompanied by hypotension and bradycardia.

Guidelines/Precautions

1. Discontinuation of clonidine ≥6 hr before surgery may result in perioperative hypertension.
2. When clonidine therapy is discontinued, rebound hypertension

may be minimized by tapered withdrawal of the drug over 2–4 days.

3. Use with caution in patients with severe coronary insufficiency, recent myocardial infarction, cerebrovascular disease, chronic renal failure, Raynaud's disease, thromboangiitis obliterans, or a history of mental depression.
4. Epidural or spinal clonidine (>10 μg/kg) may produce dose-dependent maternal and fetal bradycardia.
5. Clonidine transdermal system is contraindicated in patients with known hypersensitivity to clonidine or to any ingredient or component in the administration system.
6. Signs and symptoms of overdosage include hypotension, transient hypertension, cardiac arrhythmias, respiratory depression, and seizures. Symptomatic and supportive measures should be instituted. Tolazoline (IV 10 mg) may reverse the cardiovascular effects.

Principal Adverse Reactions

Cardiovascular: Hypotension, rebound hypertension with drug withdrawal, CHF, AV block.
Pulmonary: Mild ventilatory depression.
CNS: Depression, anxiety.
GU: Impotence, urinary retention.
GI: Nausea, vomiting, parotid pain.
Dermatologic: Rash, angioneurotic edema.

COCAINE HCL (COCAINE HCL)

Use(s): Topical anesthesia and vasoconstrictor (mucous membranes only).
Dosing: Topical, 1.5 mg/kg (1%–4% solution).
Nasal, 1–2 mL each nostril (1%–10% solution). Concentrations >4% increase potential for systemic toxic reactions. Maximum safe dose, 1.5 mg/kg.
Elimination: Plasma cholinesterase, hepatic.
How Supplied: Cocaine solvets (soluble tablets): 135 mg with lactose; topical solution: 4%, 10%; powder: 5 g, 25 g.

Pharmacology

A naturally occurring alkaloid and a topical anesthetic that stabilizes the neuronal membrane, preventing the initiation and trans-

mission of nerve impulses. Sympathetically mediated vasoconstriction occurs secondary to a block in the uptake of
catecholamines at adrenergic nerve endings. Small doses initially
produce bradycardia and a decrease in arterial pressure by central
vagal stimulation, but after moderate doses blood pressure and
heart rate increase. It stimulates the CNS, including the vomiting
center, and produces euphoria.

Pharmacokinetics

Onset of Action: <1 min.
Peak Effect: 2–5 min.
Duration of Action: 30–120 min.
Interaction/Toxicity: Causes sloughing of corneal epithelium and
raises intraocular pressure; potentiates arrhythmogenic effects of
sympathomimetics.

Guidelines/Precautions

1. Not for intraocular or IV use.
2. Sensitizes the heart to catecholamines. Concomitant use with
   epinephrine is dangerous and unnecessary.
3. In some patients, even small doses of 0.4 mg/kg may cause
   hypertension, ventricular fibrillation, and cardiac arrest.
4. Use with caution in patients with severely traumatized mucosa and sepsis in the region of proposed application.
5. High addiction potential.

Principal Adverse Reactions

Cardiovascular: Hypertension, bradyarrhythmias, tacharrhyth-
mias, ventricular fibrillation.
Pulmonary: Tachypnea, respiratory failure.
CNS: Euphoria, excitement, seizures.
Eyes: Sloughing of corneal epithelium.

COUMARIN DERIVATIVE—WAFARIN SODIUM (COUMADIN, PANWARFARIN, SOFARIN, CARFIN)

Use(s): Prophylaxis and/or treatment of venous thrombosis, pulmonary embolism; prophylaxis and/or treatment of thromboembo-

lism in patients with atrial fibrillation, dilated cardiomyopathy, prosthetic heart valves; adjunct in prophylaxis of systemic embolism after myocardial infarction.

Dosing: Initial dose: PO/IV/IM, 10–15 mg.
Daily dose: PO, 2–10 mg.
(Adjust according to prothrombin time [PT] response. 1.2–2.0 times control. Preferably for standardized reporting, adjust dosing to INR [International Normalized Ratio] of 2 to 3 for low-intensity anticoagulation and INR of 4 to 5 for high-intensity anticoagulation.)

Elimination: Renal, hepatic.

How Supplied: Tablets: 1 mg, 2 mg, 2.5 mg, 5 mg, 7.5 mg, 10 mg.
Injection: 50-mg vial with 2-mL diluent.

Pharmacology

4-Hydroxy-coumarin and its derivatives (warfarin sodium, dicumarol) depress synthesis in liver of vitamin K–dependent clotting factors II, VII, IX, and X. Warfarin sodium inhibits thrombus formation when stasis is induced. It does not have a direct effect on an established thrombus but may prevent further extension.

Pharmacokinetics

Onset of Action: IV/IM/PO 8–12 hr.
Peak Effect: IV/IM/PO, 1–5 days.
Duration of Action: IV/IM/PO, 2–10 days.
Interaction/Toxicity: Risks of hemorrhage increased with concomitant use of platelet aggregation inhibitors such as aspirin, phenylbutazone, other NSAIDs; enhanced anticoagulant effect with phenylbutazone, disulfiram, cimetidine and clofibrate; decreased effect with alcohol, antihistamines, and barbiturates.

Guidelines/Precautions

1. The oral anticoagulants have a great potential for clinically significant drug reactions. Patients should not take any drugs, including nonprescription products, without the advice of a physician or pharmacist.
2. Periodic determination of PT is essential. Monitor PT daily during the initiation of therapy, with the addition or discon-

tinuation of an interacting drug, and q4–6wk after the patient's condition is stabilized.

3. Contraindicated when risk of hemorrhage is greater than potential clinical benefits.

4. Regional anesthesia is contraindicated.

5. Effects counteracted by administration of vitamin K (PO, 2.5–10 mg with mild or no bleeding; IV, 5–50 mg with frank bleeding), fresh whole blood or fresh frozen plasma (15 mL/kg).

6. The INR takes into account the variability of each laboratory's source and preparation of tissue thromboplastin used in determining the prothrombin time ratio (patient's PT divided by control PT). The INR standardizes the prothrombin time ratio by using an intrinsic sensitivity index (ISI), which is a measure of the tissue thromboplastin (INR = PTR^{ISI}).

Principal Adverse Reactions

Hematologic: Agranulocytosis, eosinophilia, leukopenia, hemorrhage from any organ.
GI: Nausea, vomiting.
Dermatologic: Necrosis of skin, urticaria, dermatitis.
Other: "Purple toes" syndrome, neuropathy, nephropathy.

CYCLOSPORINE (SANDIMMUNE)

Use(s): Immunosuppression for organ transplantation, treatment of chronic allograft rejection in patients previously treated with other immunosupressive agents, e.g., azathioprine, treatment of severe autoimmune disease resistant to corticosteroids and other therapy.

Dosing: (organ transplantation):

Preoperative, PO: 15 mg/kg (range, 6–18 mg/kg). IV infusion: 0.5–6 mg/kg (over 2–6 hr). Administer as single dose 4–12 hours prior to transplantation.

Postoperative, PO: 15 mg/kg (range, 6–18 mg/kg) once daily for 1–2 wk. Taper by 5%/wk (over 6–8 wk) to:

Maintenance, PO: 4–10 mg/kg.

> Postoperative, IV infusion: 0.5–6 mg/kg once daily
> (Give over 2–6 hr). Switch to oral administration as
> soon as possible after surgery.

Patients receiving IV cyclosporine should be closely monitored
for allergic reactions or anaphylaxis. Appropriate equipment for
resuscitation should be readily available. Trough blood or plasma
concentrations (i.e., at 24 hr) of 250–800 or 50–300 ng/mL, respectively, as determened by radioimmunoassay (RIA), minimize
the frequency of graft rejection and cyclosporine induced adverse
effects. Concomitant corticosteroid/azathioprine therapy is recommended.

> Prednisone: PO, 2 mg/kg daily for 4 days tapered to 1
> mg/kg/day by 1 wk, 0.6 mg/kg/day by 2 wk, 0.3
> mg/kg/day by 1 mo, 0.15 mg/kg/day by 2 mo and
> thereafter as a maintenance dose. Adjustments in
> dosage of prednisone must be made according to
> the clinical situation.
>
> Azathioprine: PO, 1–2 mg/kg/day.
>
> Acute Allograft Rejection: Methylprednisolone 0.5-1
> g/day for 3 days. Maximum dose, 6 g. If rejection
> continues discontinue cyclosporine and continue
> with azathioprine and corticosteroids.

Note: numerous protocols exist and change continuously.

Elimination: Hepatic.

How Supplied: Capsules (liquid filled): 25 mg, 100 mg. Oral
solution: 100 mg/mL. Injection (concentrate for
infusion): 50 mg/mL.

Dilution for Infusion: 50 mg in 50 mL NS or D_5W (1 mg/mL).

Pharmacology

A cyclic polypeptide antibiotic, cyclosporine is a potent immunosuppressive agent produced by the fungus species *Tolypocladium
inflatum Gams*. It inhibits cell-mediated immune responses such
as allograft rejection, delayed hypersensitivity (e.g., tuberculin induced), experimental allergic encephalomyelitis, Freund's adju-
vant-induced arthritis, and graft-vs.-host disease. Cyclosporine
may also inhibit humoral immune responses. It prolongs survival
of allogenic transplants involving skin, heart, kidney, pancreas,
bone marrow, small intestine, and lung. Unlike other currently
available immunosupressive agents, cyclosporine lacks clinically

important myelosuppressive activity. Bone marrow cell counts (i.e., granulocytes, monocytes, stem cells) show only slight reductions in cell numbers with normal or enhanced stem cell proliferation. Cyclosporine produces dose-dependent and reversible hepatotoxic and nephrotoxic effects. Increased plasma renin activity may contribute to the development of hypertension. The clinical importance of its antimalarial, antineoplastic, and antischistosomal activity has not been determined.

Pharmacokinetics

Onset: PO, variable.
Peak Effect: PO, 3.5 hr (peak blood levels).
Duration: Half-life, 10–40 hr.
Interaction/Toxicity: Additive nephrotoxic effects with concomitant use of other nephrotoxic drugs, e.g., acyclovir. indomethacin, disopyramide, aminoglycoside antibiotics, amphotericin B; increased plasma concentrations of cyclosporine and elevated serum creatinine with ketoconazole, erythromycin, methotrexate, methylprednisolone, verapamil, diltiazem, acetazolamide, diclofenac; increased creatinine clearance with concomitant administration of cimetidine and ranitidine; decreased plasma concentrations of cyclosporine with warfarin, rifampin, phenytoin, phenobarbital, sulfamethazine, and trimethoprim; cyclosporine may interfere with the activity of warfarin and the elimination of methotrexate; may prolong neuromuscular blockade of nondepolarizing muscle relaxants, e.g., atracurium, vecuronium; concomitant administraiton with furosemide may result in hyperuricemia and gout; concomitant administration with potassium-sparing diuretics, e.g., spironolactone, may result in hyperkalemia; GI absorption increased by oral metoclopramide; increased incidence of gingival hyperplasia with calcium channel blockers, especially nifedipine; cyclosporine increases serum levels of digoxin and combined therapy may result in digoxin toxicity; concomitant administration with disulfiram may result in an Antabuse-type reaction (due to the alcohol content of the oral and intravenous formulations of cyclosporine).

Guidelines/Precautions

1. Use only under the supervision of a physician experienced in immunosupressive therapy and management of organ transplant patients.

2. Increases susceptibility to infections and lymphoma, especially with concomitant administration of other immunosuppressive agents.

3. Because of the risk of anaphylaxis, IV cyclosporine should be reserved for patients who are unable to tolerate the oral formulation of the drug.

4. Periodic monitoring of renal function, hepatic function, blood, or plasma cyclosporine concentrations are especially important.

5. Increased BUN and serum creatinine do not necessarily indicate that organ rejection has occurred. In patients with renal allografts, acute episodes of allograft rejection must be differentiated from nephrotoxic effects of cyclosporine. Increased serum creatinine concentrations without the usual symptoms of allograft rejection (e.g., fever, graft tenderness, or enlargement) imply cyclosporine-induced nephrotoxicity.

6. If severe intractable renal allograft rejection occurs, it is preferable to allow the kidney to be rejected and removed than to increase cyclosporine dosage to a high level in an attempt to reverse the rejection episode.

7. Increased frequency of seizures in children may be related to concomitant hypertension or high-dose corticosteroid therapy.

Principal Adverse Reactions

Cardiovascular: Hypertension, chest pain, myocardial infarction.
CNS: Headache, tremors, seizures, paresthesia, confusion, anxiety, depression, neurotoxic syndrome (cortical blindness, quadriplegia, seizures, and/or coma), possibly associated with low serum cholesterol.
GI: Nausea, vomiting, anorexia, diarrhea, constipation, peptic ulcer, hiccups, abdominal discomfort.
Hepatic: Abnormal liver function tests.
GU: Increased BUN and serum creatinine, hyperkalemia, fluid retention.
Metabolic: Hyperchloremic hyperkalemic metabolic acidosis.
Infectious Complications: Pneumonia, septicemia, abscesses, and urinary tract, viral, local, systemic fungal, skin, and wound infections.
Hematologic: Leukopenia, anemia, thrombocytopenia, lymphoma.
Allergic: Anaphylaxis.

Dermatologic: Flushing, hirsutism, gingival hyperplasia.
Other: Hyperlipidemia, hyperglycemia, hypomagnesemia, conjunctivitis, tinnitus, fever, pancreatitis, benign fibroadenoma, gynecomastia, sinusitis, aseptic necrosis, weight loss, night sweats.

DANTROLENE SODIUM (DANTRIUM)

Use(s): Treatment or prevention of malignant hyperthermia; relief of spasticity from upper motor neuron disease.
Dosing: Malignant hyperthermia:

> Treatment: IV push, 1–2 mg/kg q5–10min. (maximum 10 mg/kg; dose may be repeated), then PO, 4–8 mg/kg/day in 3 divided doses for up to 3 days after the crisis.

> Prophylaxis: Infusion, 2.5 mg/kg over 15–30 min just before induction of anesthesia, and/or PO, 4–8 mg/kg/day in 3 divided doses for 1–2 days, last dose 3 hr before anesthesia. Apropriate supportive measures (outlined later) should be instituted in conjunction with drug treatment.

> Chronic spasticity: PO, 25 mg once daily. Titrate upward to 100 mg bid or qid.

Elimination: Hepatic, renal.
How Supplied: Vials containing 20 mg dantrolene and 3000 mg mannitol to be reconstituted in 60 ml sterile water; capsules, 25 mg, 50 mg, and 100 mg.

Pharmacology

Dantrolene is a direct-acting skeletal muscle relaxant. It inhibits the release of calcium from the sarcoplasmic reticulum. Neuromuscular transmission and electrical properties of the skeletal muscle membrane are not altered. It attenuates or reverses the physiologic, metabolic, and biochemical changes associated with malignant hyperthermia crisis. Skeletal muscle weakness may interfere with ventilation and protective pharyngeal reflexes.

Pharmacokinetics

Onset of Action: PO, 1–2 hr; IV, <5 min.
Peak Effect: PO, 4–6 hr; IV, 1 hr.

Duration of Action: PO, 8–9 hr; IV, 3 hr.
Interaction/Toxicity: Combination with calcium channel blockers may produce hyperkalemia and cardiovascular collapse; hepatitis may occur with long-term use.

Guidelines/Precautions

1. Avoid combination with calcium channel blockers during management of malignant hyperthermia. May cause ventricular fibrillation and cardiovascular collapse in association with marked hyperkalemia.
2. Other supportive measures must be continued in the management of malignant hyperthermia. These include discontinuing the suspect triggering agents, attending to increased oxygen requirements, managing the metabolic acidosis, instituting cooling, and monitoring the urinary output and electrolyte balance. (See Appendix A: Malignant Hyperthermia Protocol.)
3. After a malignant hyperthermia crisis, oral or IV dantrolene should be used for up to 3 days to prevent a recurrence.
4. Monitor liver function if therapy exceeds 45 days.
5. Women more than age 35 yr have a greater risk of hepatotoxicity, especially if taking concurrent medications such as estrogens.

Principal Adverse Reactions

Cardiovascular: Tachycardia, labile blood pressure.
CNS: Drowsiness, dizziness, seizures.
GU: Hematuria, urinary frequency, incontinence.
GI: Diarrhea, constipation.
Hepatic: Fatal or nonfatal hepatitis.
Dermatologic: Rash, pruritus.
Musculoskeletal: Myalgia, backache.

DESMOPRESSIN ACETATE (DDAVP, STIMATE)

Use(s): Maintenance of hemostasis after cardiopulmonary bypass; treatment of neurogenic diabetes insipidus, hemophilia A (with factor VIII levels >5%), von Willebrand's disease (type I with factor VIII levels >5%), and primary nocturnal enuresis.

Dosing: Diabetes insipidus: Intranasal, 0.1–0.4 mL daily.
Hemophilia A/von Willebrand's disease, hemostasis after cardiopulmonary bypass: IV. 0.3 μg/kg; dilute in 50 mL sterile saline solution; give over 30 min. If plasma factor VIII level is <5%, do not rely on desmopressin.

Elimination: Renal.

How Supplied: Intranasal, 0.1 mg/mL; injection, 4 μg/mL.

Pharmacology

Desmopressin is a synthetic analogue of 8-arginine vasopressin (ADH) with antidiuretic activity. It increases the cyclic AMP content of cells in the renal tubules and collecting ducts, which increases cellular permeability to water. As a consequence, the urine becomes more concentrated. Desmopressin also releases von Willebrand's factor necessary for adequate activity of factor VIII and optimal function of platelets. It may produce elevation of blood pressure.

Pharmacokinetics

Onset of Action: IV, 15–30 min (increase in plasma factor VIII activity); intranasal, <1 hr (antidiuretic effects).

Peak Effect: IV, 90 min–3 hr (increase in plasma factor VIII activity); intranasal, 1–5 hr (antidiuretic effects).

Duration of Action: IV 6–20 hr (increase in plasma factor VIII activity); intranasal, 8–20 hr (antidiuretic effects).

Interaction/Toxicity: Water intoxication and hyponatremia; elevation of blood pressure, antidiuretic effect potentiated by chlorpropamide, carbamazepine, and clofibrate.

Guidelines/Precautions

1. Monitor fluid intake.
2. Severe allergic reaction with repeated use.
3. Use with caution in patients with hypertension and coronary artery disease.
4. Do not use in patients with type IIB or platelet-type (pseudo) von Willebrand's disease. May cause platelet aggregation and thrombocytopenia.
5. Patients should be weighed daily to check for edema.

Principal Adverse Reactions

Cardiovascular: Coronary ischemia, hypertension.
CNS: Headache.
GI: Abdominal pain, nausea.
Dermatologic: Flushing, erythema.
Other: Water intoxication, hyponatremia, rhinitis.

DEXAMETHASONE (DECADRON, HEXADROL)

Use(s): Treatment of cerebral edema, aspiration pneumonitis, bronchial asthma, myofascial trigger points, allergic reactions; prevention of rejection in organ transplantation; replacement therapy for adrenocortical insufficiency.

Dosing: Dexamethasone phosphate.

> IV/IM, 0.5–25 mg/day. Trigger point, 1–4 mg (dilute in 10 mL local anesthetic); may repeat at 1–3 wk. Intraarticular/intratissue, 1–16 mg; may repeat at 1–3 wk. Inhalation, 300 μg (3 inhalations) 3 or 4 times daily.

> Dexamethasone acetate:
> IM, 8–16 mg/day; repeat in 1–3 wk.

> Dexamethasone:
> PO, 0.75–9 mg/day. (Taper off dose if used for more than a few days.)

Elimination: Hepatic.

How Supplied: Injection—dexamethasone phosphate (IV/IM): 4 mg/mL, 10 mg/mL, 20 mg/mL. Injection—dexamethasone phosphate (IV use only): 20 mg/mL, 24 mg/mL. Injection—dexamethasone acetate (IM use only): 8 mg/mL, 16 mg/mL. Tablets—dexamethasone: 0.25 mg, 0.5 mg, 0.75 mg, 1.5 mg, 4 mg, 6 mg. Oral solution—dexamethasone: 0.1 mg/mL. Aerosol—dexamethasone phosphate: 100 μg/metered spray.

Pharmacology

A fluorinated derivative of prednisolone with potent anti-inflammatory effect. 0.75 mg is equivalent to 20 mg cortisol. At equipotent doses, dexamethasone lacks the sodium-retaining property of hydrocortisone. It may suppress the hypothalamic-pituitary-adrenal axis.

Pharmacokinetics

Onset of Action: IV/IM, few minutes.
Peak Effect: IV/IM, 12–24 hr.
Duration of Action: IV/IM, 36–54 hr.
Interaction/Toxicity: Clearance enhanced by phenytoin, phenobarbital, ephedrine, rifampin; altered response to coumarin anticoagulants; increases requirements of insulin; interacts with anticholinesterase agents (e.g., neostigmine) to produce severe weakness in patients with myasthenia gravis; potassium-wasting effects enhanced with potassium-depleting diuretics (e.g., thiazides, furosemide); diminishes response to toxoids and live or inactivated vaccines.

Guidelines/Precautions

1. Induced adrenocortical insufficiency with rapid withdrawal of dexamethasone.
2. Use with caution in patients with hypertension, CHF, thromboembolytic tendencies, hypothyroidism, cirrhosis, myasthenia gravis, peptic ulcer, diverticulitis, nonspecific ulcerative colitis, fresh intestinal anastomosis, psychosis, seizure disorders, antibiotic-resistant systemic fungal and viral infections.
3. Administration of live virus vaccines (i.e., smallpox) is contraindicated in patients receiving immunosuppressive doses.

Principal Adverse Reactions

Cardiovascular: Arrhythmias, hypertension, CHF in susceptible patients.
CNS: Seizures, increased intracranial pressure, corticosteroid psychosis.
Dermatologic: Impaired wound healing, petechiae, erythema.
Eye: Increased intraocular pressure, subcapsular cataracts.
Metabolic: Fluid retention, sodium retention, potassium depletion.
Endocrine: Secondary adrenocortical and pituitary unresponsiveness during stress, growth suppression, increased requirements for insulin.
Musculoskeletal: Myopathy, weakness, osteoporosis.
Other: Thromboembolism, diminished response to toxoids and

live or inactivated vaccines, increased susceptibility to and masking of symptoms of infection.

DIAZEPAM (VALIUM)

Use(s): Premedication, amnesia, sedative/hypnotic, induction agent, skeletal muscle relaxant, anticonvulsant, treatment of acute alcohol withdrawal and panic attacks.

Dosing: Premedication: IV/PO, 2–10 mg (0.1–0.2 mg/kg); IM, 0.4 mg/kg.

Induction: IV, 0.3–0.5 mg/kg.

Anticonvulsant: IV, 0.1–0.2 mg/kg q10–15min; maximum dose, 30 mg; PO, 2–10 mg bid to qid; PO (extended release), 15–30 mg once daily. .

Withdrawal: IV, 0.1–0.2 mg/kg q3–4h; PO, 5–10 mg tid or qid; PO (extended release), 15–30 mg once daily.

Elimination: Hepatic.

How Supplied: Tablets: 2 mg, 5 mg, 10 mg; capsule (sustained release): 15 mg; oral solution: 5 mg/mL; injection: 5 mg/mL.

Pharmacology

A benzodiazepine derivative that acts on the limbic system, thalamus, and hypothalamus, inducing calming effects. It exerts antianxiety and skeletal muscle–relaxing effects by increasing the availability of the glycine inhibitory neurotransmitter, whereas the sedative action reflects the ability of benzodiazepines to facilitate actions of the inhibitory neurotransmitter GABA. The site of action for production of anterograde amnesia has not been confirmed. Diazepam has no peripheral autonomic blocking action. It has minimal depressant effects on ventilation and circulation in the absence of other CNS depressant drugs. Prolonged recovery.

Pharmacokinetics

Onset of Action: IV <2 min; PO, 15 min–1 hr (shorter in children).

Peak Effect: IV, 3–4 min; PO, 1 hr.

Duration of Action: IV, 15 min–1 hr; PO, 2–6 hr.

Interaction/Toxicity: Sedative and circulatory depressant effect potentiated by opioids, alcohol, and other CNS depressants; elimination reduced by cimetidine; reduces requirements for volatile anesthetics; thrombophlebitis with IV administration; decreased clearance and dosage requirements in old age; effects antagonized by flumazenil; may cause neonatal hypothermia; interacts with plastic containers and administration sets, significantly decreasing bioavailability.

Guidelines/Precautions

1. Contraindicated in acute narrow-angle or open-angle glaucoma unless patients are receiving appropriate therapy.
2. Reduce dose in elderly, high-risk, or hypovolemic patients, patients with limited pulmonary reserve, and with concomitant use of other sedatives or narcotics.
3. Slow injection through large veins to reduce thrombophlebitis.
4. Return of drowsiness may occur 6–8 hr after dose because of enterohepatic recirculation.
5. Treat overdose with supportive measures and flumazenil (slow IV, 0.2–1 mg).
6. IM route is painful and results in slow erratic absorption.
7. Do not mix or dilute with other solutions or drugs.

Principal Adverse Reactions

Cardiovascular: Bradycardia, hypotension.
Pulmonary: Respiratory depression.
CNS: Drowsiness, ataxia, confusion, depression, paradoxical excitement.
GU: Incontinence.
Dermatologic: Rash.
Other: Venous thrombosis and phlebitis at site of injection, dry mouth, hypotonia, hyperthermia.

DIGOXIN (LANOXIN)

Use(s): Inotropic agent; treatment of heart failure and supraventricular arrhythmias.

Dosing: Adults: Loading: IV/PO, 0.5–1 mg in divided doses. (Give 50% of loading dose as first dose, then 25% fractions at 4–8 hr intervals until an adequate therapeutic response is attained, toxic effects occur or the total digitalizing dose has been administered. Monitor clinical response before each additional dose; maintenance: IV/PO, 0.125–0.5 mg daily; dosages should be individualized.

Elderly adults (>65 yr): PO, 0.125 mg daily as maintenance dose; frail or small patients may require less.

Children >2 yr: PO loading: 0.02–0.06 mg/kg divided q8h for 24 hr; IV loading: 0.015–0.035 mg/kg divided q8h for 24 hr; maintenance: PO/IV, 25%–35% loading dose daily divided q12h.

Children 1 mo–2 yr: PO loading: 0.035–0.06 mg/kg divided q8h for 24 hr; IV loading: 0.03–0.05 mg/kg divided q8h for 24 hr; maintenance: PO/IV, 25%–35% loading dose daily divided q12h.

Full-term neonates: PO loading: 0.025–0.035 mg/kg divided q8h for 24 hr; IV loading: 0.02–0.03 mg/kg divided q8h for 24 hr; maintenance: PO/IV, 25%–35% loading dose daily divided q12h.

Premature neonates: PO loading: 0.02–0.03 mg/kg divided q8h for 24 hr; IV loading: 0.015–0.025 mg/kg divided q8h for 24 hr; maintenance: PO/IV, 0.25–0.35 loading dose daily divided q12h. Therapeutic drug levels are 0.5–2 ng/mL in adults and 1.1–1.7 ng/mL in neonates and infants. Higher levels may be required for heart rate control in atrial fibrillation. *Note:* Therapeutic levels do not exclude toxicity.

Elimination: Renal.

How Supplied: Tablets: 0.125 mg, 0.25 mg, 0.5 mg; capsules (Lanoxicaps): 0.05 mg, 0.1 mg, 0.2 mg; oral solution 0.05 mg/mL; injection: 0.1 mg/mL, 0.25 mg/mL.

Pharmacology

This glycoside composed of a sugar and a cardenolide has a direct inotropic effect via inhibition of the sodium-potassium adenosine triphosphatase (ATPase) ion transport system. It has an indirect vagomimetic effect, with decreased activity of the SA node and prolonged conduction through the AV node. Digoxin increases contractility and decreases myocardial oxygen consumption in the failing heart.

Pharmacokinetics

Onset of Action: IV, 5–30 min; PO, 30 min–2 hr.
Peak Effect: IV, 1–4 hr; PO, 2–6 hr.
Duration of Action: IV/PO, 3–4 days (digitalized patients).
Interaction/Toxicity: Enhanced toxicity in hypokalemia, hypo-magnesemia, hypercalcemia; increased serum levels with calcium channel blockers (e.g., verapamil, nifedipine, diltiazem), es-molol, quinidine, amiodarone, flecainide, captopril, benzodiaz-epines, anticholinergics, oral aminoglycosides, erythromycin; re-sistance in atrial fibrillation associated with hypermetabolism (e.g., hyperthyroidism); succinylcholine may cause arrhythmias in digitalized patients; overdosage may cause complete heart block, AV dissociation, ventricular tachycardias, or fibrillation.

Guidelines/Precautions

1. Decreased dosage requirements in patients with impaired re-nal function, and the elderly.
2. Monitor serum potassium and digoxin levels. To allow for equilibration of digoxin between serum and tissue, determine serum digoxin levels at least 4 hr after an IV dose and 6 hr after an oral dose.
3. Contraindicated in ventricular fibrillation.
4. Use of synchronized cardioversion in a patient with digitalis toxicity should be avoided because it may initiate ventricular fibrillation.
5. Steady-state levels may take as long as 7 days.
6. Use with succinylcholine may precipitate arrhythmias.
7. Use caution when switching from lanoxicaps to standard tab-lets because of increased bioavailability.
8. Digoxin toxicity may manifest with anorexia, nausea, vomit-ing, cardiac arrhythmias, headache, drowsiness, hyperkale-mia, normokalemia, or hypokalemia. Discontinue digoxin, monitor serum electrolyte and glycoside concentrations, and initiate supportive and symptomatic treatment. Digoxin-immune Fab is a specific antidote. Give in approximate

equimolar quantities as total dose of glycoside absorbed. Empirical dose of 800 mg (20 40-mg vials) of digoxin-immune Fab is adequate to treat most life-threatening toxicity in adults and children. Small children should be monitored closely for fluid overload when this large dose is used.

Principal Adverse Reactions

Cardiovascular: Wide range of arrhythmias, AV block.
CNS: Headache, psychosis, confusion.
GI: Nausea, vomiting, diarrhea.
Other: Gynecomastia.

DIPHENHYDRAMINE HCL (BENADRYL)

Use(s): Antiemetic, antivertigo, treatment of allergic reactions; adjuvant use in the treatment of anaphylaxis, symptomatic treatment of drug-induced extrapyramidal reactions.
Dosing: PO, 25–50 mg (0.3–0.5 mg/kg) q6–8h.
  IV/IM, 10–50 mg (0.2–0.5 mg/kg).
  Maximum daily dose, 400 mg.
Elimination: Hepatic.
How Supplied: Tablets: 25 mg, 50 mg; capsules: 25 mg, 50 mg; oral solution: 12.5 mg/5 mL; injection: 10 mg/mL, 50 mg/mL.

Pharmacology

This is a histamine H_1 receptor antagonist with anticholinergic and sedative effects. It partially inhibits vasodilator effects of histamine on peripheral vascular smooth muscle. Diphenhydramine should be employed in anaphylactic reactions as adjunctive therapy only after epinephrine and other lifesaving measures have been used.

Pharmacokinetics

Onset of Action: IV, few minutes; PO, <15 min.
Peak Effect: IV 1–3 hr; PO, 2 hr.
Duration of Action: IV/PO, <7 hr.
Interaction/Toxicity: Anticholinergic effects potentiated by MAO inhibitors; additive sedative effect with alcohol, hypnotics, sedatives, and tranquilizers.

Guidelines/Precautions

1. Children are at increased risk for experiencing paradoxical CNS stimulant effects (restlessness, insomnia, tremors, euphoria, seizures).
2. Use with caution in patients with narrow-angle glaucoma, increased intraocular pressure, seizure disorders bowel or bladder neck obstruction, lower respiratory diseases, including asthma.
3. Contraindicated in newborn or premature infants.

Principal Adverse Reactions

Cardiovascular: Hypotension, palpitation, extrasystoles.
Pulmonary: Wheezing, tightness of chest.
CNS: Sedation, confusion, blurred vision, tinnitus, seizures, tremors.
GU: Urinary frequency, urinary retention.

DOBUTAMINE HCL (DOBUTREX)

Use(s): Inotrope, pharmacologic stress test in coronary artery disease.
Dosing: Infusion, 0.5–30 μg/kg/min.
Elimination: Hepatic.
How Supplied: Injection: 12.5 mg/mL.
Dilution for Infusion: 500 mg in 500 mL D_5W or NS solution (1 mg/mL).

Pharmacology

A β_1-adrenergic agonist that increases myocardial rate and force of contraction. In therapeutic doses, it has mild β_2- and α_1-adrenergic receptor agonist effects and decreases peripheral and pulmonary vascular resistance. Dobutamine does not stimulate release of endogenous norepinephrine and does not act on dopaminergic receptors.

Pharmacokinetics

Onset of Action: 1–2 min.
Peak Effect: 1–10 min.

Duration of Action: <10 min.
Interaction/Toxicity: Less effective with β-blockers; use with nitroprusside results in higher cardiac output and lower pulmonary
wedge pressure; bretylium potentiates effects of dobutamine and
may result in arrhythmias; inactivated in alkaline solutions; increased risk of supraventricular and ventricular arrhythmias with
use of volatile anesthetics.

Guidelines/Precautions

1. Arrhythmias and hypertension at high doses. Higher risk of
   dangerous arrhythmias with use of volatile anesthetics.
2. Contraindicated in idiopathic hypertrophic subaortic stenosis
   (IHSS).
3. Do not mix with sodium bicarbonate, furosemide, or other
   alkaline solutions.
4. In patients with atrial fibrillation and rapid ventricular rate, a
   digitalis or other heart rate–controlling preparation should be
   instituted before therapy with dobutamine is commenced.
5. Correct hypovolemia as fully as possible before or during
   treatment.
6. Drug contains sodium bisulfite and may trigger hypersensitivity reactions.

Principal Adverse Reactions

Cardiovascular: Hypertension, tachycardia, arrhythmias, angina.
Pulmonary: Shortness of breath.
CNS: Headache.
Other: Phlebitis at injection site.

DOPAMINE HCL (INTROPIN)

Use(s): Inotropic agent, vasoconstrictor, diuresis in cardiac or
acute renal failure.
Dosing: Infusion: 1–50 μg/kg/min.
Elimination: Hepatic.
How Supplied: Injection: parenteral concentrate for infusion,
40, 80, and 160 mg/mL; premixed solution in 5% dextrose, 80
mg/100 mL, 160 mg/100 mL, 320 mg/100 mL.
Dilution for Infusion: 400 mg in 250 mL D_5W or NS solution
(1600 μg/mL).

Pharmacology

A naturally occurring catecholamine that acts directly on α-, β_1-, and dopaminergic receptors and indirectly by releasing norepinephrine from its storage sites. At low doses ($1-3$ µg/kg/min) specifically increases blood flow to the renal, mesenteric, coronary, and cerebral beds by activating the dopamine receptors. A rise in glomerular filtration rate and increased sodium excretion accompany the increase in renal blood flow. Infusion of dopamine at $2-10$ µg/kg/min stimulates β_1-adrenergic receptors in the heart, causing an increase in myocardial contractility, stroke volume, and cardiac output. Doses >10 µg/kg/min stimulate α-adrenergic receptors causing an increase in peripheral vascular resistance, decreased renal blood flow, and an increased potential for arrhythmias.

Pharmacokinetics

Onset of Action: $2-4$ min.
Peak Effect: $2-10$ min.
Duration of Action: <10 min.
Interaction/Toxicity: Increased risk of supraventricular and ventricular arrhythmias with use of volatile anesthetics; possible necrosis in patients with occlusive vascular disease; inactivated in alkaline solutions; concomitant use with phenytoin may cause seizures, severe hypotension, and bradycardia.

Guidelines/Precautions

1. Infuse into large vein. Extravasation may cause sloughing and necrosis. Treat by local infiltration of phentolamine ($5-10$ mg in 10 mL NS).
2. Correct hypovolemia as fully as possible before or during treatment.

Principal Adverse Reactions

Cardiovascular: Arrhythmias, angina, AV block, hypotension, hypertension, vasoconstriction.
Pulmonary: Dyspnea.
CNS: Headache, anxiety.
GI: Nausea and vomiting.
Dermatologic: Piloerection.
Other: Gangrene of extremities with prolonged period of high doses.

DOXACURIUM CHLORIDE (NUROMAX)

Use(s): Nondepolarizing muscle relaxant.
Dosing: IV (paralyzing), 0.05–0.08 mg/kg.
 Pretreatment/maintenance, 0.005–0.01 mg/kg.
Elimination: Renal.
How Supplied: Injection: 1 mg/mL.

Pharmacology

A long-acting nondepolarizing neuromuscular blocking agent. It binds competitively to cholinergic receptors on the motor end plate and antagonizes the action of acetylcholine, resulting in a block of neuromuscular transmission.

Doxacurium is 2.5–3 times more potent than pancuronium. The time of onset and duration are similar to those of pancuronium at comparable doses. The drug has no clinically significant hemodynamic effects. Histamine release rarely occurs.

Pharmacokinetics

Onset of Action: <4 min.
Peak Effect: 3–9 min.
Duration of Action: 30–160 min.
Interaction/Toxicity: Potentiated by prior administration of succinylcholine, volatile anesthetics, aminoglycoside antibiotics, small doses of local anesthetics, loop diuretics, magnesium, lithium, phenytoin, ganglionic blocking drugs, hypothermia, hypokalemia, respiratory acidosis; recurrent paralysis with quinidine, enhanced neuromuscular blockade in patients with myasthenia gravis or inadequate adrenocortical function; effects antagonized by anticholinesterase inhibitors such as neostigmine, edrophonium, pyridostigmine; increased resistance or reversal of effects with use of carbamazepine, phenytoin, and in patients with burn injury and paresis; incompatible with alkaline solutions with a pH > 8.5, such as barbiturate solutions.

Guidelines/Precautions

1. Monitor response with peripheral nerve stimulator to minimize risk of overdosage.
2. Reverse effects with anticholinesterases such as pyridostigmine bromide, neostigmine, or edrophonium in conjunction with atropine or glycopyrrolate. Neostigmine (0.05 mg/kg) is

more effective than edrophonium (1 mg/kg) in antagonizing moderate to deep levels of neuromuscular block.
3. Pretreatment doses may induce a degree of neuromuscular blockade sufficient to cause hypoventilation in some patients.

Principal Adverse Reactions

Cardiovascular: Hypotension, flushing, ventricular fibrillation, myocardial infarction.
Pulmonary: Hypoventilation, apnea, bronchospasm.
CNS: Depression.
GU: Anuria.
Dermatologic: Rash, urticaria.
Musculoskeletal: Inadequate block, prolonged block.

DOXAPRAM HCL (DOPRAM)

Use(s): Respiratory stimulant.
Dosing: Slow IV: 0.5–1.5 mg/kg; repeat in 5 min; Maximum
           dose, 2 mg/kg.
         Infusion: 5 mg/min until satisfactory respiratory re-
           sponse is obtained, then 1–3 mg/min; maximum
           dose, 4 mg/kg.
Elimination: Hepatic.
How Supplied: Injection: 20 mg/ml.
Dilution for Infusion: 250 mg in 250 mL D_5W or NS solution
(1 mg/mL).

Pharmacology

A respiratory stimulant with action mediated through the peripheral carotid chemoreceptors. As dosage level is increased, the central respiratory centers in the medulla are stimulated, with progressive stimulation of other parts of the brain and spinal cord. Stimulant action is manifested by an increase in tidal volume associated with a slight increase in respiratory rate. Doxapram may produce a pressor response because of the release of catecholamines and improved cardiac output. This is more marked in hypovolemic patients. Although opiate-induced respiratory depression is antagonized, the analgesic effect is not affected. Stimulation of respiration is short lived and is useful only in patients with drug-induced postanesthesia respiratory depression or apnea other than that caused by muscle relaxant drugs.

Pharmacokinetics

Onset of Action: 20–40 sec.
Peak Effect: 1–2 min.
Duration of Action: 5–12 min.
Interaction/Toxicity: Additive pressor effect in patients receiving sympathomimetics or MAO inhibitors; may mask residual effects of muscle relaxants; increased risk of arrhythmias in patients receiving volatile anesthetics; precipitate formation with alkaline solutions such as thiopental, bicarbonate, and aminophylline.

Guidelines/Precautions

1. Because of benzyl alcohol content, do not use in newborns.
2. Contraindicated in patients with epilepsy, convulsive disorders, mechanical disorders of ventilation (e.g., mechanical obstruction, muscle paresis, flail chest, pneumothorax, acute bronchial asthma, pulmonary fibrosis, conditions resulting in restriction of chest walls, muscles of respiration, or alveolar expansion). Also contraindicated in patients with evidence of head injury, cerebral vascular accident, significant cardiovascular impairment, severe hypertension, or known hypersensitivity to the drug.
3. It is neither an antagonist to muscle relaxant nor a specific narcotic antagonist. Adequacy of airway and oxygenation must be assured before administration.
4. Maintain close observation of patient for 1 hr after patient has been fully alert, because narcosis may recur.
5. Do not use in conjunction with mechanical ventilation.
6. Use with caution in patients with hypermetabolic states.
7. Because of myocardial sensitization to catecholamines, delay administration for at least 10 min after discontinuation of volatile anesthetics.

Principal Adverse Reactions

Cardiovascular: Hypertension, chest pain, tachycardia, bradycardia, arrhythmias.
Pulmonary: Cough, tachycardia, laryngospasm, bronchospasm, hiccups.

CNS: Seizures, hyperactivity, headache, disorientation, clonus, pupillary dilation.
GU: Urinary retention, spontaneous voiding, proteinuria.
GI: Nausea, vomiting, desire to defecate.
Hematologic: Decreased hemoglobin level, hematocrit, red blood cell (RBC) count, and leukopenia.

DROPERIDOL (INAPSINE)

Use(s): Antiemetic, premedication, neuroleptic.
Dosing: Antiemetic: IV, 0.625–2.5 mg (15 μg/kg).
Premedication: IV/IM, 2.5–10 mg.
Neuroleptanesthesia: IV, 0.2 mg/kg, with fentanyl, 4 μg/kg.
Elimination: Hepatic, renal.
How Supplied: Injection: 2.5 mg/mL, combination with fentanyl citrate (Innovar). Injection: droperidol, 2.5 mg/mL, with fentanyl citrate, 50 μg/mL.

Pharmacology

A butyrophenone derivative. It interferes with CNS transmission at dopamine, noradrenaline, serotonin, and GABA synaptic sites. Droperidol produces marked tranquilization and sedation, inducing a state of mental detachment and indifference while maintaining a state of reflex alertness. Antiemetic effects are caused by receptor blockade in the chemoreceptor trigger zone. The drug has an α_1-adrenergic antagonist action that may produce a decrease in systemic vascular resistance and blood pressure. It may be combined with fentanyl to produce neuroleptanalgesia and anesthesia.

Pharmacokinetics

Onset of Action: IM/IV, 3–10 min.
Peak Effect: IM/IV, 30 min.
Duration of Action: IM/IV, 2–4 hr.
Interaction/Toxicity: Potentiates other CNS depressants; reduces pressor and arrhythmogenic effects of epinephrine; may induce extrapyramidal symptoms.

Guidelines/Precautions

1. Rule out hypotension as a cause or result of emesis before administering droperidol.
2. Contraindicated in patients with Parkinson's disease. Extrapyramidal reactions may consist of dystonic reactions, feelings of motor restlessness (akathisia), and parkinsonian signs and symptoms. Therapy should include discontinuation of droperidol or reduction in dosage and treatment with an anticholinergic antiparkinsonian agent (e.g., benztropine or trihexyphenidyl) or diphenhydramine (IV/PO, 25 mg). Maintenance of an adequate airway should be instituted if necessary.
3. Prolonged CNS depression may occur with neuroleptanalgesia.

Principal Adverse Reactions

Cardiovascular: Hypotension, tachycardia.
Pulmonary: Laryngospasm, bronchospasm.
CNS: Extrapyramidal symptoms, drowsiness, hyperactivity.

D-TUBOCURARINE CHLORIDE (TUBOCURARINE CHLORIDE)

Use(s): Nondepolarizing muscle relaxant.
Dosing: Paralyzing: IV, 0.3–0.6 mg/kg.
      Pretreatment/maintenance: IV, 0.05–0.1 mg/kg.
      Infusion: 1–6 μg/kg/min.
Elimination: Renal, hepatic.
How Supplied: Injection: 3 mg/mL.
Dilution for Infusion: 15 mg in 100 mL D_5W (0.15 mg/mL).

Pharmacology

D-Tubocurarine is an intermediate-acting, nondepolarizing neuromuscular-blocking agent. It competes for cholinergic receptors at the motor end plate. The hypotension associated with clinical doses is secondary to autonomic ganglion blockade and release of histamine. Repeated doses may have a cumulative effect.

Pharmacokinetics

Onset of Action: <2 min.
Peak Effect: 2–6 min.
Duration of Action: 25–90 min.
Interaction/Toxicity: Effects potentiated by volatile anesthetics, aminoglycoside antibiotics, local anesthetics, diuretics, magnesium, lithium, ganglion-blocking drugs, respiratory acidosis, hypokalemia; effects antagonized by anticholinesterase inhibitors such as neostigmine, edrophonium, and pyridostigmine; resistance with concomitant use of phenytoin and in patients with burn injury and paresis; reduces MAC requirement for volatile anesthetics.

Guidelines/Precautions

1. Monitor response with peripheral nerve stimulator to minimize risk of overdosage.
2. Use with caution in patients with history of bronchial asthma and anaphylactoid reactions.
3. Reverse effects with anticholinesterases such as pyridostigmine bromide, neostigmine, or edrophonium in conjunction with atropine or glycopyrrolate.
4. Pretreatment doses may induce a degree of neuromuscular blockade sufficient to cause hypoventilation in some patients.

Principal Adverse Reactions

Cardiovascular: Hypotension, bradycardia, arrhythmias.
Pulmonary: Respiratory depression, apnea.
Musculoskeletal: Inadequate block, prolonged block.
Dermatologic: Rash, urticaria.

EDROPHONIUM CHLORIDE (TENSILON, ENLON, REVERSOL)

Use(s): Reversal of nondepolarizing muscle relaxants, diagnostic assessment of myasthenia gravis.
Dosing: Reverse neuromuscular blockade: slow IV, 0.5–1.0 mg/kg; maximum dose, 40 mg (with atropine, 0.015 mg/kg, or glycopyrrolate, 0.01 mg/kg).

Assessment of myasthenia/cholinergic crisis: slow IV, 1
mg q1–2min until change in symptoms; maximum
dose, 10 mg. IM, 10 mg.

Elimination: Hepatic, renal.
How Supplied: Injection: 10 mg/mL.

Pharmacology

This short-acting quaternary ammonium anticholinesterase agent
inhibits the hydrolysis of acetylcholine by competitively binding
acetylcholinesterase. The buildup of acetylcholine facilitates the
transmission of impulses across the neuromuscular junction. In
myasthenia gravis there is improved skeletal muscle tone in
conditions of low acetylcholine levels and increased skeletal
muscle weakness in conditions of cholinergic crisis. Cholinergic
stimulation may be useful in terminating supraventricular
tachyarrhythmias. When used for reversal of neuromuscular
blockade, the muscarinic cholinergic effects (bradycardia, salivation) are prevented by concurrent use of atropine or glycopyrrolate.

Pharmacokinetics

Onset of Action: IV, 30–60 sec; IM, 2–10 min.
Peak Effect: IV, 1–5 min.
Duration of Action: IV 5–20 min; IM, 10–40 min.
Interaction/Toxicity: Does not antagonize and may prolong the
phase 1 block of depolarizing muscle relaxants such as succinylcholine; antagonizes the effects of nondepolarizing muscle
relaxants such as tubocurarine, atracurium, vecuronium, and
pancuronium; antagonism of neuromuscular blockade is reduced by aminoglycoside antibiotics, corticosteroids, magnesium,
hypothermia, hypokalemia, and respiratory and metabolic acidosis.

Guidelines/Precautions

1. Contraindicated in patients with peritonitis or mechanical obstruction of the intestines or urinary tract.
2. Use with caution in patients with bradycardia, bronchial
   asthma, cardiac arrhythmias, or peptic ulcer.
3. Edrophonium overdosage may induce a cholinergic crisis
   characterized by nausea, vomiting, bradycardia or tachycar-

dia, excessive salivation and sweating, bronchospasm, weakness, and paralysis.
4. Treatment of a cholinergic crisis includes discontinuation of edrophonium and administration of atropine (10 µg/kg IV q3–10min until muscarinic symptoms disappear) and, if necessary, pralidoxime (15 mg/kg IV over 2 min) for reversal of nicotinic symptoms.
5. Due to the brief duration of action of edrophonium, neostigmine or pyridostigmine are generally preferred for reversal of the effects of nondepolarizing muscle relaxants.

Principal Adverse Reactions

Cardiovascular: Bradycardia, tachycardia, AV block, nodal rhythm, hypotension.
Pulmonary: Increased oral, pharyngeal and bronchial secretions, bronchospasm, respiratory depression.
CNS: Seizures, dysarthria, headaches.
Eye: Lacrimation, miosis, visual changes.
GI: Nausea, emesis, flatulence, increased peristalsis.
Dermatologic: Rash, urticaria.
Allergic: Allergic reactions, anaphylaxis.

EPHEDRINE SULFATE (EPHEDRINE SULFATE)

Use(s): Vasopressor, bronchodilator.
Dosing: IV, 5–20 mg (100–200 µg/kg); IM 25–50 mg; PO, 25–50 mg q3–4h.
Elimination: Hepatic, renal.
How Supplied: Injection, 25 mg/mL, 50 mg/mL; capsules, 25 mg, 50 mg; oral solution, 20 mg/5 mL.

Pharmacology

This drug is a noncatecholamine sympathomimetic with mixed direct and indirect actions. It is resistant to metabolism by MAO and catechol-O-methyltransferase (COMT), resulting in prolonged duration of action. Ephedrine increases cardiac output, blood pressure, and heart rate by α- and β-adrenergic stimulation. It increases coronary and skeletal blood flow and produces bronchodilation by stimulation of β_2-receptors.

Pharmacokinetics

Onset of Action: IV, almost immediate; IM few minutes.
Peak Effect: IV, 2–5 min; IM, <10 min.
Duration of Action: IV/IM, 10–60 min.
Interaction/Toxicity: Increased risk of arrhythmias with volatile anesthetic agents; potentiated by tricyclic antidepressants; increases MAC of volatile anesthetics.

Guidelines/Precautions

1. Tolerance may develop, but temporary cessation of the drug restores its original effectiveness.
2. Use cautiously in patients with hypertension and ischemic heart disease.
3. Has unpredictable effect in patients in whom endogenous catecholamines are depleted.
4. May produce an unacceptable degree of CNS stimulation, resulting in insomnia.

Principal Adverse Reactions

Cardiovascular: Hypertension, tachycardia, arrhythmias.
Pulmonary: Pulmonary edema.
CNS: Anxiety, tremors.
Metabolic: Hyperglycemia, transient hyperkalemia, and then hypokalemia.
Dermatologic: Necrosis at site of injection.

EPINEPHRINE HCL (ADRENALINE, EPINEPHRINE)

Use(s): Inotrope, bronchodilator, prolongation of duration of local anesthetics, treatment of allergic reactions, after intubation and infectious croup, resuscitation.
Dosing: Cardiac arrest: 0.5–1 mg IV bolus (5–10 mL or 0.1 mL/kg of 1:10,000 solution); repeat q5min as necessary.
Inotropic support: Infusion, 2–20 μg/min (0.1–1.0 μg/kg/min).

Anaphylaxis/severe asthma: Adults, 0.1–0.5 mg SC or
IM (0.1–0.5 ml 1:1000 solution); children, 0.01
mg/kg SC or IM (0.01 mL/kg 1:1000 solution), not
to exceed 0.5 mg.

SC doses may be repeated at 10- to 15-min intervals in patients
with anaphylactic shock and at 20-min to 4-hr intervals in patients
with asthma.

Bronchodilator/croup therapy inhalation: Nebulization
with O_2, 1% (1:100) epinephrine *or* 2.25% racemic
epinephrine; dilute 1 mL in 3 mL NS solution; give
1–3 inhalations and repeat after 5 min if necessary;
administer treatments q2–6h; no <30 min between
treatments. (Children: 0.5% [1:200] epinephrine or
1.25% racemic epinephrine. Dilute 0.5 mL in 1.5
mL NS solution. Give q2–6h.)

Metered aerosol: 160–250 µg (1 inhalation); repeat
once if necessary after at least 1 min; subsequent doses
should not be administered for at least 4 hr.*

Prolongation of local/epidural anesthesia: 1:200,000 to
1:100,000 solution mixed with local anesthetic; (0.1
mg epinephrine diluted in 20 mL local anesthetic gives
1:200,000 solution, or 5 µg/mL.)

Prolongation of spinal anesthesia: 0.1–0.4 mg
(0.1–0.4 mL 1:1000 solution) added to anesthetic
spinal fluid mixture.

Elimination: Enzymatic degradation (hepatic, renal, and GI[3]
tract).

How Supplied: Injection: 0.01 mg/mL (1:100,000), 0.1 mg/mL
(1:10,000), 0.5 mg/mL (1:2,000), 1 mg/mL (1:1,000); solution
for nebulization: 1% epinephrine, 1.25% racemic epinephrine,
2.25% racemic epinephrine; aerosol: 1600 µg/metered spray, 200
µg/metered spray, 250 µg/metered spray.

Dilution for Infusion: 3 mg in 250 mL D_5W or NS solution (12
µg/mL).

Pharmacology

An endogenous catecholamine that activates both α- and β-adrenergic receptors. At therapeutic parenteral doses, the prominent ef-

*Rebound effect with obstruction may follow initial clearing of airway. Monitor
patient closely.

fects are on β adrenergic receptors. There is increased myocardial contractility and heart rate, relaxation of the smooth muscle of the bronchial tree, dilation of skeletal muscle vasculature, and a decrease in total peripheral resistance. At higher doses, α-adrenergic effects predominate, and there is an increase in total peripheral resistance. Epinephrine decreases the rate of absorption of local anesthetics. It prolongs the duration of anesthesia, thereby decreasing the risk of systemic toxicity.

Pharmacokinetics

Onset of Action: IV, immediate; SC 6–15 min; inhalation, 3–5 min.
Peak Effect: IV within 3 min.
Duration of Action: IV, 5–10 min; inhalation/SC, 1–3 hr.
Interaction/Toxicity: Ventricular arrhythmias, (increased risk with use of volatile anesthetics, especially halothane); reduction of renal blood flow and urinary outflow; enhanced effect with tricyclic antidepressants and bretylium.

Guidelines/Precautions

1. Use with digitalis or volatile anesthetics may result in arrhythmias. The 50% effective dose (ED_{50}) of epinephrine in NS solution per 20 min needed to produce ≥3 premature ventricular contractions in adults: 1.25 MAC halothane 1.5 μg/kg, 1.25 MAC enflurane 3.5 μg/kg, 1.25 MAC isoflurane 6.5 μg/kg. The ED_{50} of epinephrine in 0.5% lidocaine: 1.25 MAC halothane 3.7 μg/kg in adults and 7.8–15 μg/kg in children.
2. Use with caution in patients with cardiovascular disease, hypertension, diabetes, and hyperthyroidism.
3. Contraindicated for local anesthesia of end organs (digits, penis, ears).
4. If IV access is not available, the drug may be injected via an endotracheal tube.

Principal Adverse Reactions

Cardiovascular: Hypertension, tachycardia, arrhythmias, angina.
Pulmonary: Pulmonary edema.
CNS: Anxiety, headache, cerebrovascular hemorrhage.
Dermatologic: Necrosis at site of injection.
Metabolic: Hyperglycemia, transient hyperkalemia, hypokalemia.

ERGONOVINE MALEATE (ERGOTRATE)

Use(s): Treatment of postpartum uterine atony and bleeding; involution of the uterus.
Dosing: IV/IM, 0.2 mg (may require repeated doses).
       PO, 0.2−0.4 mg q6−12h for 48 hr.
Elimination: Hepatic.
How Supplied: Injection, 0.2 mg/mL; tablets, 0.2 mg.

Pharmacology

This ergot alkaloid stimulates contractions of uterine and vascular smooth muscle. It increases contractile frequency and tone of the uterine musculature. Ergonovine produces vasoconstriction (mainly of capacitance vessels), increased central venous pressure, and elevated blood pressure.

Pharmacokinetics

Onset: IV, 40 sec; IM, 7−8 min; PO, 10 min.
Peak Effect: IV <5 min; IM <1 hr.
Duration: IV, 45 min; IM, 3−6 hr.
Interaction/Toxicity: Vasoconstriction potentiated by sympathomimetics (e.g., ephedrine, phenylephrine).

Guidelines/Precautions

1. Administration in the second or third stage of labor before delivery of the placenta may lead to captivation of the placenta.
2. Use cautiously in patients with preeclampsia, hypertension, or cardiac disease.
3. Avoid in patients with peripheral vascular disease.
4. Uterine contractions may continue for ≥3 hr after injection.
5. IV administration has a higher incidence of side effects and should be used in emergency situations only.
6. Severe cramping is evidence of effectiveness of oral doses but may justify reduction in dosage.

Principal Adverse Reactions

Cardiovascular: Hypertension, tachycardia.
CNS: Cerebrovascular accidents, seizures.

GI: Nausea and vomiting.
Eye: Retinal detachment.

ESMOLOL HCL (BREVIBLOC)

Use(s): Treatment of supraventricular tachyarrhythmias, perioperative and intraoperative hypertension.
Dosing: IV loading: 500 µg/kg/min. (Give over 1 min.)
Infusion: 50–200 µg/kg/min (if no therapeutic effect, repeat loading dose at intervals of 5 min and titrate maintenance dose upward in increments of 25–50 µg/kg/min).
Infusion doses >200 µg/kg/min provide little added benefit.
Elimination: Esterases (in cytosol of RBCs).
How Supplied: Injection: 10 mg/mL, 250 mg/mL.
Dilution for Infusion: 5 g in 500 mL D_5W (10 mg/mL). 10 mg/mL vials do not need to be diluted.

Pharmacology

A cardioselective β-blocker with rapid onset and short duration of action. The drug is hydrolyzed by RBC esterases. It produces negative inotropic and chronotropic effects. At high doses, selectivity for β_1-adrenergic receptors usually diminishes, and inhibition of β_2-receptors of bronchial and vascular smooth muscle will occur.

Pharmacokinetics

Onset of Action: 1–2 min.
Peak Effect: 5 min.
Duration of Action: 10–20 min.
Interaction/Toxicity: Potentiates myocardial depression produced by inhaled or injected anesthetics; may unmask the direct negative inotropic effect of ketamine, incompatible with sodium bicarbonate.

Guidelines/Precautions

1. Use with caution in patients with AV heart block or cardiac failure not caused by tachycardia and in patients with chronic obstructive airway disease.

2. May mask signs of hypoglycemia in diabetes mellitus.
3. Excessive myocardial depression may be treated with IV atropine (1–2 mg), IV isoproterenol (0.02–0.15 µg/kg/min), IV glucagon (1–5 mg), or a transvenous cardiac pacemaker.
4. May enhance the actions of nondepolarizing neuromuscular blocking agents such as tubocurarine, gallamine, metocurine, and pancuronium.
5. After achieving adequate heart rate and blood pressure control, transfer to an alternative antiarrhythmic or antihypertensive such as propranolol, verapamil, or digoxin. Reduce infusion rate of esmolol by 50% 30 min after the first dose of alternative agent. Discontinue esmolol after second dose if pressure and rate control have been attained.

Principal Adverse Reactions

Cardiovascular: Hypotension, bradycardia.
Pulmonary: Bronchospasm.
CNS: Confusion, depression.
GU: Urinary retention.
GI: Nausea, vomiting.
Dermatologic: Erythema, edema at infusion site.

ETHACRYNIC ACID (EDECRIN)

Use(s): Diuretic; treatment of hypertension, increased intracranial pressure, edema associated with congestive heart failure, hepatic cirrhosis, and nephrotic syndrome; differential diagnosis of acute oliguria.
Dosing: Slow IV, 0.5–1 mg/kg.
PO, 50–200 mg/day (children 25 mg/day initial dose and adjust in increments of 25 mg).
Elimination: Renal.
How Supplied: Powder for injection, 50 mg/vial in 50 mL vials for reconstitution; tablets, 25 mg, 50 mg.

Pharmacology

This loop diuretic inhibits reabsorption of sodium and chloride ions primarily in the medullary portion of the ascending limb of the loop of Henle. It inhibits reabsorption of sodium to a greater proportion than most other diuretics and may be effective in patients with significant degrees of renal insufficiency.

Pharmacokinetics

Onset of Action: IV, <5 min; PO, 30 min.
Peak Effect: IV, 15–30 min; PO, 2 hr.
Duration of Action: IV, 2 hr; PO, 6–8 hr.
Interaction/Toxicity: Potassium loss increases likelihood of digitalis toxicity and enhances effects of muscle relaxants; has additive effects with other diuretics; potentiates carbonic anhydrase inhibitors; coadministration of aminoglycosides and cisplatin may increase potential for ototoxicity.

Guidelines/Precautions

1. Do not use to treat acute oliguria caused by decreased intravascular volume.
2. Monitor fluid and electrolyte values periodically.
3. Use with caution in patients with hearing impairment or cirrhosis.
4. May predispose patients to digitalis glycoside toxicity because of hypokalemia.
5. Do not give SC or IM because of pain and irritation at site.

Principal Adverse Reactions

Cardiovascular: Hypotension.
CNS: Headaches, confusion.
GI: Anorexia, malaise, diarrhea, abdominal discomfort, bleeding.
Metabolic: Hyperuricemia.
Special Senses: Deafness, tinnitus, vertigo, blurred vision.
Other: Rash, fever, chills, hematuria.

ETIDOCAINE HCL (DURANEST)

Use(s): Regional anesthesia.
Dosing: Infiltration/peripheral nerve block, 50–400 mg (1% solution).

Epidural, 100–300 mg (1% or 1.5% solution).

Caudal, 100–300 mg (10–30 mL 1% solution; children, 0.4–0.7 mL/kg for L2–T10 level of anesthesia.

Maximum safe dose, 3 mg/kg without epinephrine, 4 mg/kg with epinephrine. Solutions containing preservatives should not be used for epidural or caudal block.

Elimination: Hepatic.

How Supplied: Injection: 1% solution with or without epinephrine, 1:200,000; 1.5% solution with epinephrine, 1:200,000.

Pharmacology

An aminoamide and a long-acting local anesthetic. It stabilizes neuronal membrane by inhibiting the ionic fluxes required for the initiation and conduction of impulses. Etidocaine produces a profound degree of motor blockade and abdominal muscle relaxation when used for peridural analgesia. Toxic blood levels may cause seizures and cardiovascular collapse secondary to a decrease in peripheral vascular resistance and direct myocardial depression. Vasoconstrictor agents decrease rate of absorption and prolong duration of action.

Pharmacokinetics

Onset of Action: Infiltration, 3–5 min; epidural, 5–15 min.

Peak Effect: Infiltration, 5–15 min; epidural, 15–20 min.

Duration of Action: Infiltration, 2–3 hr (with epinephrine 3–7 hr); epidural, 3–5 hr.

Interaction/Toxicity: Reduced clearance with concomitant use of β-blocking agents, cimetidine; seizures, respiratory, and circulatory depression at high plasma levels; benzodiazepines increase seizure threshold; duration of local or regional anesthesia prolonged by vasoconstrictor agents, e.g., epinephrine.

Guidelines/Precautions

1. Do not use for spinal anesthesia.
2. Because of profound motor blockade, not recommended for epidural anesthesia in normal delivery.

3. Use with caution in patients with hypovolemia, severe CHF, shock, and all forms of heart block.
4. Contraindicated in patients with hypersensitivity to amide-type local anesthetics.
5. Benzodiazepines increase seizure threshold.
6. Use for paracervical block can be associated with fetal bradycardia.
7. Toxic plasma levels, e.g., from accidental intravascular injection, may cause cardiopulmonary collapse and seizures. Premonitory signs and symptoms manifest as numbness of the tongue and circumoral tissues, metallic taste, restlessness, tinnitus, and tremors. Support of circulation (IV fluids, vasopressors, defibrillation) and securing a patent airway (ventilate with 100% oxygen) are paramount. Thiopental (1–2 mg/kg IV), midazolam (0.02–0.04 mg/kg IV), or diazepam (0.1 mg/kg IV) may be used for prophylaxis and/or treatment of seizures.
8. The level of sympathetic blockade (bradycardia with block above T5) determines the degree of hypotension (often heralded by nausea and vomiting) following epidural or intrathecal etidocaine. Fluid hydration (10–20 mL/kg NS or lactated Ringer's solution), vasopressor agents, e.g., ephedrine, and left uterine displacement in pregnant patients may be used for prophylaxis and/or treatment. Administer atropine to treat bradycardia.
9. Epidural or caudal injections should be avoided when the patient has hypovolemic shock, septicemia, infection at the injection site or coagulopathy.

Principal Adverse Reactions

Cardiovascular: Bradycardia, hypotension.
Pulmonary: Respiratory depression.
CNS: Euphoria, tinnitus, seizures.
Allergic: Urticaria, edema, anaphylactoid symptoms.
Epidural/Caudal: High spinal, loss of bladder and bowel control, loss of perineal sensation and sexual function, persistent motor sensory and/or autonomic (sphincter control) deficit.

ETOMIDATE (AMIDATE)

Use(s): Induction of anesthesia.
Dosing: IV, 0.1–0.4 mg/kg.
Elimination: Hepatic.
How Supplied: Injection: 2 mg/mL.

Pharmacology

A nonbarbiturate hypnotic without analgesic activity. Therapeutic doses have minimal effect on myocardial metabolism, cardiac output, and peripheral or pulmonary circulation. Etomidate reduces intracranial and intraocular pressure. Myoclonic movements occur in about one third of patients during induction and are caused by disinhibition of subcortical suppression of extrapyramidal activity. Adrenocortical suppression, which may occur after a single induction dose, lasts 4–8 hr and is caused by etomidate-induced inhibition of 11β-hydroxylase.

Pharmacokinetics

Onset of Action: 30–60 sec.
Peak Effect: 1 min.
Duration of Action: 3–10 min.
Interaction/Toxicity: Effects potentiated by other sedatives, narcotics; venous pain and myoclonus on rapid injection.

Guidelines/Precautions

1. Use with caution in patients with focal epilepsy.
2. Use large veins. Pain more likely if injected into small veins.
3. Myoclonus reduced by premedication with benzodiazepine or opioid.

Principal Adverse Reactions

Cardiovascular: Hypotension, hypertension, arrhythmias.
Pulmonary: Hyperventilation, hypoventilation, laryngospasm, hiccups.
CNS: Myoclonus, tonic movements, eye movements.
GI: Nausea or vomiting.

Endocrine: Adrenocortical suppression.
Other: Thrombophlebitis.

FAMOTIDINE (PEPCID)

Use(s): Peptic ulcer disease, pathologic hypersecretory states, prophylaxis against acid pulmonary aspiration or allergic reaction.
Dosing: IV, 20 mg q12h (dilute in 10 mL NS solution; inject over 2 min).
    PO, 20 mg twice daily or 40 mg at bedtime.
Elimination: Renal.
How Supplied: Tablets, 20 mg, 40 mg; powder for oral suspension, 40 mg/5 mL when reconstituted; injection, 10 mg/mL.

Pharmacology

This competitive inhibitor of histamine H_2 receptors suppresses acid concentration and volume of gastric secretion. Gastric emptying and exocrine pancreatic functions are not affected. It does not have any cumulative effect with repeated doses.

Pharmacokinetics

Onset of Action: PO, within 1 hr; IV, <30 min.
Peak Effect: PO, 1–4 hr; IV, 30 min–3 hr.
Duration of Action: PO/IV, 10–12 hr.
Interaction/Toxicity: Bioavailability enhanced by food and decreased by antacids.

Guidelines/Precautions

Reduce dosage in patients with renal impairment.

Principal Adverse Reactions

Cardiovascular: Palpitations, hypotension.
Pulmonary: Bronchospasm.
CNS: Tinnitus, fatigue, dizziness, depression, paresthesia, headache.
GI: Nausea, vomiting, diarrhea.
Musculoskeletal: Musculoskeletal pain, arthralgia.
Hematologic: Thrombocytopenia.

FENTANYL (SUBLIMAZE)*

Use(s): Analgesia, anesthesia.
Dosing: Analgesia: IV/IM, 0.7–2 µg/kg; oral transmucosal, 5–20 µg/kg.

Induction: IV, 5–30 µg/kg; infusion, 0.05–0.2 µg/kg/min.

Epidural: Bolus, 1–2 µg/kg; infusion, 25–60 µg/hr (0.5–0.7 µg/kg/hr).

Spinal: Bolus, 0.1–0.4 µg/kg.

Brachial plexus block: Add 1–2 µg/kg fentanyl to 40 mL local anesthetic.

Patient-controlled analgesia:

IV: Bolus, 15–75 µg; infusion, 15–25 µg/hr; lockout interval, 3–10 min.

Epidural: Bolus, 4–8 µg; infusion, 6 µg/hr; lockout interval, 10 min.

Transdermal: base dose on prior 24-hr analgesic requirements. 60 mg IM morphine dose = 360 mg; PO morphine dose = 100 µg/hr transdermal fentanyl dose.

Elimination: Hepatic.
How Supplied: Injection: 50 µg/mL; transdermal: 25 µg/hr, 50 µg/hr, 75 µg/hr, 100 µg/hr.
Dilution for Infusion: IV: 500 µg in 100 mL NS (5 µg/mL). Epidural: 200–500 µg in 100 mL local anesthetic or (preservative-free) NS solution (2–5 µg/mL).

Pharmacology

This phenylpiperidine derivative is a potent opioid agonist. As an analgesic, fentanyl is 75–125 times more potent than morphine. The rapid onset and short duration of action reflects the greater lipid solubility of fentanyl compared with morphine. Depression of ventilation is dose dependent and may last longer than the analgesia. Cardiovascular stability is maintained even in large doses when used as a sole anesthetic. Fentanyl is combined with droperidol to produce neuroleptanalgesia.

*For epidural/intrathecal precautions, see Alfentanil, Guidelines/Precautions, items 5 and 6, pp. 4–5.

Pharmacokinetics

Onset of Action: IV, within 30 sec; IM, <8 min; epidural/spinal, 4–10 min; transdermal, 12–18 hr; oral transmucosal, 10–60 min.
Peak Effect: IV, 5–15 min; IM, <15 min; epidural/spinal, <30 min; oral transmucosal, 15–60 min.
Duration of Action: IV, 30–60 min; IM, 1–2 hr; epidural/spinal, 4–8 hr; transdermal, 3 days; oral transmucosal, 1–2 hr.
Interaction/Toxicity: Circulatory and ventilatory depressant effects potentiated by narcotics, sedatives, volatile anesthetics, nitrous oxide; ventilatory depressant effects potentiated by amphetamines, MAO inhibitors, phenothiazines, and tricyclic antidepressants; analgesia enhanced by α_2-agonists, e.g., clonidine, epinephrine; muscle rigidity in higher dose range sufficient to interfere with ventilation.

Guidelines/Precautions

1. Reduce doses in elderly, hypovolemic, high-risk patients, and with concomitant use of sedatives and other narcotics. Incremental doses should be determined from effect of initial dose.
2. Narcotic effects reversed by naloxone (≥0.2–0.4 mg IV). Duration of reversal may be shorter than duration of narcotic action.
3. High doses may produce a naloxone sensitive–increased muscle tone and rigidity.
4. Crosses the placental barrier, and usage in labor may produce depression of respiration in the neonate. Resuscitation may be required; have naloxone available.

Principal Adverse Reactions

Cardiovascular: Hypotension, bradycardia.
Pulmonary: Respiratory depression, apnea.
CNS: Dizziness, blurred vision, seizures.
GI: Nausea, emesis, delayed gastric emptying, biliary tract spasm.
Musculoskeletal: Muscle rigidity.

FLECAINIDE ACETATE (TAMBOCOR)

Use(s): Treatment of documented life-threatening ventricular arrhythmias, such as sustained ventricular tachycardia.

Dosing: PO: 100–200 mg q12h. Keep trough levels <0.2–1.0 μg/mL.

Elimination: Renal, hepatic.

How Supplied: Tablets: 100 mg (IV not available for general clinical use in the United States).

Pharmacology

A fluorinated analogue of procainamide, flecainide is a class 1C antiarrhythmic. It produces dose-related decrease in intracardiac conduction in all parts of the heart, with the greatest effect on the His-Purkinje system (H-V conduction). This results in QRS complex widening and prolonged QT interval. Pacing threshold is increased by flecainide. Although it does not usually alter heart rate, it exerts a moderate negative inotropic effect and reduced ejection fraction. Flecainide's use should be reserved for treatment of documented, life-threatening arrhythmias after failure of conventional therapy.

Pharmacokinetics

Onset of Action: <1 hr.

Peak Effect: 2–4 hr.

Duration of Action: 12–27 hr (half-life).

Interaction/Toxicity: Additive negative inotropic effects with β-adrenergic blockers, calcium channel blockers; excretion decreased by alkalinization and increased by acidification; altered effects with hypokalemia or hyperkalemia; may cause new or worsened arrhythmias.

Guidelines/Precautions

1. Use with caution in patients with a history of CHF, myocardial dysfunction, and sick sinus syndrome, and those with permanent pacemakers or temporary pacing electrodes.
2. Do not administer to patients with existing poor endocardial pacing thresholds or nonprogrammable pacemakers unless suitable pacing rescue is available.

3. Correct preexisting hypokalemia or hyperkalemia before administration.
4. Increased urinary pH decreases and decreased urinary pH increases flecainide excretion.
5. Potassium status may alter the drug's effect.
6. Initiate therapy in hospital and monitor rhythm. Do not increase dosage more frequently than once q 4 days, because optimal effect may not be achieved during the first 2–3 days of therapy.

Principal Adverse Reactions

Cardiovascular: Arrhythmias, new or worsened CHF, AV block, sinus bradycardia, sinus arrest, palpitations, chest pain.
Pulmonary: Dyspnea, bronchospasm.
CNS: Dizziness, blurred vision, headache, tremor, somnolence, tinnitus.
GI: Nausea, vomiting, constipation, diarrhea, abdominal pain.
GU: Polyuria, urinary retention.
Hematologic: Leukopenia, thrombocytopenia.

FLUMAZENIL (MAZICON)

Use(s): Diagnostic and therapeutic reversal of benzodiazepine receptor agonists.
Dosing: IV bolus, 0.2–1 mg (4–20 μg/kg) at rate of 0.2 mg/min, titrate to patient response (may repeat at 20-min intervals; maximum single dose of 1 mg; maximum total dose of 3 mg in any one hour).

Infusion, 30–60 μg/min (0.5–1 μg/kg/min), maximum total dose of 3 mg in any one hour. Lack of patient response at 5 minutes after cumulative dose above 5 mg implies that the major cause of sedation is unlikely to be due to benzodiazepines.
Elimination: Hepatic.
How Supplied: Injection, 0.1 mg/mL.
Dilution for Infusion: IV, 3 mg in 50 mL D_5W or NS (60 μg/mL).

Pharmacology

Flumazenil is a benzodiazepine receptor antagonist with little or no agonist activity. It competitively inhibits the activity at the benzodiazepine recognition site on the GABA/benzodiazepine receptor complex in the central nervous system. It reverses sedation, respiratory depression, and psychomotor effects of benzodiazepines (e.g., midazolam, diazepam, flurazepam, lorazepam). Hypoventilation and amnesia may not be fully reversed. Doses and plasma levels required to reverse each agonist depends on the particular benzodiazepine and the residual plasma level; e.g., higher doses are required to reverse lorazepam than diazepam (a less potent benzodiazepine). The administration of flumazenil to patients given agonists is remarkably free of cardiovascular effects, unlike opioid reversal with naloxone. Re-sedation may occur and is more common with larger doses of benzodiazepine (>20 mg of midazolam), long procedures (>60 minutes) and use of neuromuscular blocking agents. Flumazenil does not affect the central nervous system effects of drugs affecting GABA-ergic neurons by means other than the benzodiazepine receptor (including ethanol, barbiturates, or general anesthetics) and does not reverse the effects of opioids. It produces withdrawal symptoms (seizures, emergent confusion, and agitation) in the presence of physical dependence.

Pharmacokinetics

Onset of Action: 1–2 min.
Peak Effect: 2–10 min.
Duration of Action: 45–90 min (variable depends on benzodiazepine plasma concentration).
Interaction/Toxicity: Reversal of sedation; precipitation of benzodiazepine withdrawal (agitation, seizures, cardiac arrhythmias); increased risk of seizures in patients with concurrent tricyclic antidepressant poisoning; may provoke panic attacks in patients with a history of panic disorders.

Guidelines/Precautions

1. The reversal of benzodiazepine effects may be associated with the onset of seizures in certain high-risk populations. Possible risk factors include concurrent major sedative-hypnotic drug

withdrawal, recent therapy with repeated doses of parenteral benzodiazepines, myoclonic jerking or seizure activity prior to flumazenil administration in overdose cases, or concurrent tricyclic antidepressant poisoning.

2. Flumazenil is not recommended in cases of serious tricyclic antidepressant poisoning. Such patients should be allowed to remain sedated (with ventilatory and circulatory support as needed) until the signs of antidepressant toxicity have subsided.

3. Treat convulsions associated with flumazenil administration with benzodiazepines, phenytoin, or barbiturates. Because of the presence of flumazenil, higher than usual doses of benzodiazepines may be required.

4. Patients who have responded to flumazenil should be carefully monitored (up to 120 min) for re-sedation, respiratory depression, or other residual benzodiazepine effects, since the duration of action of the benzodiazepine may exceed that of flumazenil. Overdose cases should always be monitored until the patients are stable and re-sedation is unlikely. The availability of flumazenil does not decrease the need for prompt detection of hypoventilation and the ability to effectively intervene by establishing an airway or assisting ventilation.

5. Necessary measures should be instituted to secure airway, ventilation and IV access prior to administering flumazenil. On arousal, patients may attempt to withdraw endotracheal tubes and/or IV lines as the result of confusion and agitation following awakening.

6. Do not use flumazenil until the effects of neuromuscular blockade have been fully reversed.

7. To minimize pain and inflammation at the injection site, administer flumazenil in a large vein. Local irritation may occur following extravasation.

Principal Adverse Reactions

Cardiovascular: Arrhythmias (atrial, nodal, ventricular extrasystoles), tachycardia, bradycardia, hypertension, angina, flushing.
CNS: Reversal of sedation, seizures, agitation, emotional lability.
GI: Nausea, vomiting.
Other: Pain at injection site, thrombophlebitis, rash, shivering.

FLURAZEPAM HCL (DALMANE)

Use(s): Premedication, sedative/hypnotic.
Dosing: PO, 15–30 mg.
Elimination: Hepatic.
How Supplied: Capsules: 15 mg, 30 mg.

Pharmacology

This benzodiazepine acts on the limbic system, thalamus, and hypothalamus. It exerts antianxiety and skeletal muscle–relaxing effects by increasing the availability of the glycine inhibitory neurotransmitter, whereas the sedative action reflects the ability of benzodiazepines to facilitate actions of the inhibitory neurotransmitter GABA. The site of action for production of anterograde amnesia has not been confirmed. It has no peripheral autonomic blocking action and minimal depressant effects on ventilation and circulation in the absence of other CNS-depressant drugs. An active metabolite, desalkylflurazepam has a half-life of 50–100 hr.

Pharmacokinetics

Onset of Action: 15 min.
Peak Effect: 30–60 min.
Duration of Action: 7–8 hr.
Interaction/Toxicity: CNS and circulatory effects potentiated by alcohol, sedatives, narcotics, volatile anesthetics; elimination reduced by cimetidine.

Guidelines/Precautions

1. Reduce dose or use a shorter-acting benzodiazepine in elderly, hypovolemic, or high-risk patients and with concomitant use of narcotics or other sedatives.
2. Not for use in children <15 yr.

Principal Adverse Reactions

Cardiovascular: Palpitations, chest pain, hypotension.
Pulmonary: Shortness of breath, respiratory depression.
CNS: Drowsiness, dizziness, ataxia, dissociation.
GI: Abdominal pain, constipation, nausea, vomiting.

FUROSEMIDE (LASIX)

Use(s): Diuretic; treatment of hypertension, pulmonary edema, increased intracranial pressure, edema associated with congestive heart failure, hepatic cirrhosis, and nephrotic syndrome; differential diagnosis of acute oliguria.

Dosing: Adults: Slow IV/IM, 5–40 mg (give IV dose slowly over 1–2 min), administer high-dose parenteral therapy as a controlled infusion (dilute in D_5W or NS solution) at a rate not exceeding 4 mg/min; PO, 20–160 mg daily. (Up to 600 mg/day with severe edema.)

Children: Slow IV/IM, 0.1–1.0 mg/kg; PO, 1–2 mg/kg daily.

Elimination: Renal.

How Supplied: Injection, 10 mg/mL; tablets, 20 mg, 40 mg, 80 mg; oral solution, 10 mg/mL, 40 mg/5 mL.

Pharmacology

An anthranilic acid derivative, this loop diuretic inhibits reabsorption of sodium and chloride ions primarily in the medullary portion of the loop of Henle. It is the diuretic of choice in acute fluid overload, such as CHF. Furosemide may reduce pulmonary wedge pressure even before a diuresis has occurred. It is useful in patients with resistant fluid retention, and in those with chronic renal insufficiency who require diuretic therapy, and as an adjunct in the management of hypertension. The drug decreases intracranial pressure by mobilizing edema fluid and interfering with sodium transport in glial tissue. Its CNS effects are not influenced by alterations in the blood-brain barrier in contrast to mannitol.

Pharmacokinetics

Onset of Action: IV, 5–15 min; PO, 30 min–1 hr.

Peak Effect: IV, 20–60 min; PO, 1–2 hr.

Duration of Action: IV, 2 hr; PO, 6–8 hr.

Interaction/Toxicity: Ototoxicity associated with rapid injection of large doses; severe renal impairment in concomitant therapy with aminoglycoside antibiotics, ethacrynic acid; reduces clearance of salicylates and lithium; potentiates antihypertensive gan-

glionic or peripheral adrenergic blocking drugs; induced hypokalemia predisposes to digitalis toxicity and potentiates action of
nondepolarizing muscle relaxants; decreased effects with coadministration of indomethacin or other NSAIDs.

Guidelines/Precautions

1. Do not use to treat acute oliguria caused by decreased intravascular volume.
2. Periodically monitor fluid and electrolyte values.
3. Use with caution in patients with liver disease. It may precipitate hepatic encephalopathy.
4. May produce a phototoxicity allergic reaction 1–2 weeks after sun exposure.

Principal Adverse Reactions

Cardiovascular: Orthostatic hypotension.
CNS: Tinnitus, hearing loss, vertigo, paresthesia.
GU: Urinary bladder spasm.
GI: Pancreatitis, nausea, vomiting, diarrhea, oral and gastric
irritation.
Hematologic: Thrombocytopenia, neutropenia, aplastic anemia.
Metabolic: Hyperglycemia, hyperuricemia, hypokalemia, hy-
pochloremic alkalosis.
Allergic: Photosensitivity, pruritus.

GALLAMINE TRIETHIODIDE (FLAXEDIL)

Use(s): Nondepolarizing muscle relaxant.
Dosing: IV paralyzing: 1–1.5 mg/kg.
       Pretreatment/maintenance: 0.1–0.3 mg/kg.
Elimination: Renal (unchanged).
How Supplied: Injection: 20 mg/mL (for IV use only).

Pharmacology

A long-acting, nondepolarizing neuromuscular blocking agent that
acts by competing for cholinergic receptors at the motor end plate.
It increases heart rate, mean arterial pressure, and cardiac output
by a selective cardiac vagal blockade, activation of the sympathetic nervous system, and inhibition of catecholamine reup-

take. Gallamine does not release histamine or block autonomic ganglia.

Pharmacokinetics

Onset of Action: 1–2 min.
Peak Effect: 3–5 min.
Duration of Action: 25–90 min.
Interaction/Toxicity: Effects potentiated by prior administration of succinylcholine, volatile anesthetics, aminoglycoside antibiotics, local anesthetics, loop diuretics, magnesium, lithium, ganglionic blocking drugs, hypothermia, hypokalemia, and respiratory acidosis; enhanced neuromuscular blockade will occur in patients with myasthenia gravis or inadequate adrenocortical function; effects antagonized by anticholinesterase inhibitors such as neostigmine, edrophonium, and pyridostigmine; increased resistance or reversal of effects with use of theophylline and in patients with burn injury and paresis.

Guidelines/Precautions

1. Monitor response with peripheral nerve stimulator to minimize risk of overdosage.
2. Contraindicated in patients with myasthenia gravis and impaired renal function.
3. Reverse effects with anticholinesterases such as neostigmine, edrophonium, or pyridostigmine bromide in conjunction with atropine or glycopyrrolate.
4. Pretreatment doses may produce a degree of neuromuscular blockade sufficient to cause hypoventilation in some patients.

Principal Adverse Reactions

Cardiovascular: Tachycardia, arrhythmias, hypotension.
Pulmonary: Hypoventilation, apnea.
Musculoskeletal: Inadequate block, prolonged block.

GLUCAGON (GLUCAGON)

Use(s): Treatment of hypoglycemia, β-blocker overdose; inotropic agent.

Dosing: Hypoglycemia: IV/IM/SC, 0.5–1 mg.
            Inotrope, IV: Bolus, 1–5 mg; infusion, 20 mg/hr.
Elimination: Renal, hepatic.
How Supplied: Vials containing 1 mg, 10 mg dry powder for reconstitution.
Dilution for Infusion: Dilute to 1 mg/mL with supplied diluent. If dose used is >2 mg, dilute with sterile water.

Pharmacology

Glucagon is a single-chain polypeptide hormone produced by α-cells of the pancreas. It acts to convert liver glycogen to glucose. In the heart, it enhances the formation of cyclic AMP but unlike catecholamines does not act via β-receptors. It increases myocardial contractility and heart rate even in the presence of β-adrenergic blockade.

Pharmacokinetics

Onset: <5 min.
Peak Effect: 5–20 min.
Duration: 10–30 min.
Interaction/Toxicity: Paradoxical hypoglycemia, hypokalemia; potentiates hypoprothrombinemic effects of anticoagulants.

Guidelines/Precautions

1. In treatment of hypoglycemic shock, liver glycogen must be available. Parenteral glucose must be given because release of insulin may subsequently cause hypoglycemia.
2. Use cautiously in patients with history of insulinoma or pheochromocytoma.
3. Rapid IV administration may cause a decrease in blood pressure.

Principal Adverse Reactions

Cardiovascular: Hypertension, hypotension.
Pulmonary: Respiratory distress.
CNS: Dizziness, lightheadedness.
GI: Nausea and vomiting.
Dermatologic: Urticaria.
Metabolic: Hypoglycemia, hyperglycemia.

GLYCOPYRROLATE (ROBINUL)

Use(s): Premedication, vagolysis, blockade of muscarinic effects of anticholinesterases, adjunctive therapy in treatment of bronchospasm and peptic ulcer.

Dosing: Premedication/vagolysis: IV/IM/SC, 0.1–0.2 mg. Children: IV/IM/SC, 4–6 μg/kg. PO, 50 μg/kg.

Reversal of neuromuscular blockade: IV, 0.01 mg/kg with anticholinesterase neostigmine, 0.05 mg/kg IV, or pyridostigmine, 0.25 mg/kg IV (0.2 mg for each 1 mg of neostigmine or 5 mg of pyridostigmine).

Bronchospasm: 0.4–0.8 mg q8h; dilute to 2–3 mL with NS solution and deliver by compressed air nebulizer.

Peptic ulcer/GI disorders: PO, 1–2 mg tid or qid.

Elimination: Renal, hepatic.

How Supplied: Injection, 0.2 mg/mL; tablets, 1 mg, 2 mg.

Pharmacology

Glycopyrrolate is a semisynthetic, quaternary ammonium, anticholinergic. Because of its highly polar nature, it resists passage across the blood-brain barrier. It inhibits action of acetylcholine by reversibly combining with muscarinic cholinergic receptors. Thus, it diminishes volume and free acidity of gastric secretions and controls excessive pharyngeal, tracheal, and bronchial secretions. Glycopyrrolate also relaxes bronchial smooth muscle, inhibits GI tone and motility, reduces tone of lower esophageal sphincter, and raises intraocular pressure by pupillary dilation. It antagonizes muscarinic symptoms (e.g., bronchorrhea, bronchospasm, bradycardia, intestinal hypermotility) induced by cholinergic drugs such as anticholinesterases. It is devoid of sedative effects.

Pharmacokinetics

Onset: IV, <1 min; IM/SC, 15–30 min; inhalation, 3–5 min. PO, 1 hr.

Peak Effect: IV, 5 min; IM/SC, 30–45 min; inhalation, 1–2 hr.

Duration of Action: IV: Vagal blockade, 2–3 hr; antisialogogue effect, 7 hr.

PO: Vagal blockade, 8–12 hr.

Inhalation: Vagal blockade, 3–6 hr.

Interaction/Toxicity: Mental confusion, especially in elderly persons; poorly absorbed orally.

Guidelines/Precautions

1. Use with great caution in patients with glaucoma, asthma, coronary artery disease, urinary bladder neck, pyloric or intestinal obstruction.
2. May accumulate and produce systemic effects with multiple dosing by inhalation.

Principal Adverse Reactions

Cardiovascular: Tachycardia (high doses), bradycardia (low doses), palpitation.
CNS: Headache, confusion, dizziness.
GU: Urinary hesitancy and retention.
GI: Nausea, vomiting.
Dermatologic: Urticaria.
Eye: Increased intraocular tension.

HALOPERIDOL (HALDOL, HALPERON)

Use(s): Tranquilizer; antipsychotic.
Dosing: IM haloperidol lactate, 2–5 mg (do not administer IV);
IM haloperidol decanoate (for chronically psychotic patients), give 10–15 times the daily oral dose (interval between doses, 4 wk) (do not administer IV.).
PO, 0.5–5 mg bid or tid. (children, 0.05–0.15 mg/kg/day).
Elimination: Hepatic.
How Supplied: Injection haloperidol lactate: 5 mg/mL; injection haloperidol decanoate, 50 mg/mL, 100 mg/mL; tablets, 0.5 mg, 1 mg, 2 mg, 5 mg, 10 mg, 20 mg; oral concentrate, 2 mg/mL.

Pharmacology

This butyrophenone derivative reduces dopaminergic neurotransmission in the CNS and the anxiety accompanying psychosis. Haloperidol is less effective against acute situational anxiety such as that present in the preoperative period. It has slight anticholinergic, α-adrenergic and ganglionic blocking effects.

Pharmacokinetics

Onset of Action: IM, 10–30 min; PO, 1–2 hr.
Peak Effect: IM, 30–45; min PO, 2–4 hr.
Duration of Action: 12–38 hr (half-life).
Interaction/Toxicity: Neuroleptic malignant syndrome; encephalopathic syndrome with coadministration of lithium; extrapyramidal reactions; may lower the seizure threshold; blocks vasopressor activity of epinephrine; potentiates anesthetics, opiates, alcohol.

Guidelines/Precautions

1. Extrapyramidal reactions may consist of dystonic reactions, feelings of motor restlessness (akathisia), and parkinsonian signs and symptoms. Dystonic reactions occur more frequently in children, whereas parkinsonian symptoms predominate in geriatric patients. Therapy should include discontinuation of haloperidol or reduction in dosage and treatment with an anticholinergic antiparkinsonian agent (e.g., benztropine, trihexyphenidyl) or diphenhydramine (IV/PO, 25 mg). Maintenance of an adequate airway should be instituted if necessary.
2. Phenylephrine or norepinephrine should be used to treat haloperidol-induced hypotension. Epinephrine may paradoxically further lower the blood pressure.
3. Use cautiously in geriatric patients, patients with glaucoma, prostatic hypertrophy, and seizure disorders, and children with acute illnesses (e.g., chickenpox, measles).
4. Neuroleptic malignant syndrome, a rare side effect, may be treated symptomatically and with dantrolene.
5. Contraindicated in Parkinson's disease.

Principal Adverse Reactions

Cardiovascular: Tachycardia, hypotension, hypertension.
Pulmonary: Laryngospasm, bronchospasm.
CNS: Extrapyramidal reaction, tardive dyskinesia.
GI: Hypersalivation, diarrhea, nausea, and vomiting.
Metabolic: Hyperglycemia, hypoglycemia, hyponatremia.
Eyes: Retinopathy, visual disturbance.

HEPARIN SODIUM (HEPARIN SODIUM)

Use(s): In vitro anticoagulant for blood samples drawn for laboratory purposes; anticoagulation during cardiopulmonary bypass; prophylaxis and treatment of venous, arterial, and intracardiac thrombosis, pulmonary embolism, atrial fibrillation with embolization; diagnosis and treatment of disseminated intravascular coagulation.

Dosing: IV flush: 10–100 units.

        Cardiopulmonary bypass: IV, 350–450 units/kg; maintain activated clotting time (ACT) of 400–480 sec.

        Low-dose thrombosis prophylaxis: 5000 units SC 2 hr before surgery, then q12h.

        Full-dose continuous IV therapy: Loading IV, 5000 units (children, 50 units/kg IV drip), then infusion, 20,000–40,000 units over 24 hr (children, 100 units/kg IV q4h, or 20,000 units/m^2/24 hr). Dilute infusion in 1 L NS solution.

        Full-dose intermittent IV therapy: Loading, 10,000 units IV then 5,000–10,000 units IV q4–6h.

        Full-dose SC therapy: Loading, 5,000 units IV and 10,000–20,000 units SC, then 8,000–10,000 units SC q8h or 15,000–20,000 SC units q12h.

Do not administer heparin IM.

Elimination: Hepatic.

How Supplied: Injection: 1000 units/mL, 2500 units/mL, 5000 units/mL, 7500 units/mL, 10,000 units/mL, 20,000 units/mL, 40,000 units/mL; lock flush solution: 10 units/mL, 100 units/mL; premixed infusion: In dextrose solution, 40 units/mL, 50 units/mL, 100 units/mL; in sodium chloride solution, 2 units/mL, 50 units/mL, 100 units/mL.

Dilution for Infusion: 25,000 units in 250 mL D$_5$W or NS (100 units/mL).

Pharmacology

This mucopolysaccharide organic acid is present endogenously in the liver and granules of mast cells and basophils. Heparin is obtained from beef lung and porcine intestinal mucosa. It combines with antithrombin III (heparin cofactor), inhibits thrombosis by inactivating activated factors IX, X, XI, and XII, inhibiting the conversion of prothrombin to thrombin. It also forms complexes with thrombin, resulting in thrombin inactivation, and prevents the formation of a stable fibrin clot by inhibiting the activation of fibrin-stabilizing factor.

Pharmacokinetics

Onset of Action: IV, immediate; SC, 20–30 min.
Peak Effect: SC, 2–4 hr.
Duration of Action: 1–3 hr (half-life) dose-dependent.
Interaction/Toxicity: Increased risk of bleeding with coadministration of platelet aggregation inhibitors such as aspirin, indomethacin, ibuprofen, dipyridamole, and hydroxychloroquine; reduced effect with digitalis, propranolol, and tetracyclines, nicotine or antihistamines; increased resistance to therapy in fever, thrombosis, thrombophlebitis, myocardial infarction, cancer, and postsurgical patients.

Guidelines/Precautions

1. Monitor activated partial thromboplastin time (APTT) or ACT for therapeutic effects. Usually APTT is 1.5–2 times control when fully anticoagulated. Perform periodic platelet counts, hematocrits, and tests for occult blood in stool and urine during the entire course of heparin therapy.
2. Contraindicated in patients with severe thrombycytopenia, thrombocytopenia induced with acute heparin therapy, or uncontrollable active bleeding not caused by disseminated intravascular coagulation.
3. IV route avoids erratic absorption of IM or SC dosing.

Principal Adverse Reactions

Hematologic: Hemorrhage, thrombocytopenia.
GI: Elevated liver enzyme levels.
Dermatologic: Erythema, necrosis at site of SC injection.
Other: Osteoporosis, priapism, hypersensitivity.

HETASTARCH (HESPAN)

Use(s): Plasma volume expander.
Dosing: IV, 250–1000 mL; maximum dose, 1500 mL (20 mL/kg)/day.
Elimination: Renal (molecules <40,000 daltons).
How Supplied: 500 ml IV infusion bottles of 6% hetastarch in 0.9% sodium chloride.

Pharmacology

This artificial colloid consists of polysaccharides with an average molecular weight of 450,000 daltons. It is composed almost entirely of amylopectin. The colloidal properties approximate those of human albumin. IV infusion results in expansion of plasma volume slightly in excess of the volume infused, which decreases from this maximum over the succeeding 24–36 hr. The expansion of plasma volume may improve the hemodynamic status for ≥24 hr. Hetastarch has antigenic properties. It does not generally interfere with blood typing or crossmatching.

Pharmacokinetics

Onset of Action: Immediate.
Peak Effect: Few minutes (after end of infusion).
Duration of Action: 24–36 hr (expansion of plasma volume in excess of volume infused).
Interaction/Toxicity: Large volumes may alter the coagulation mechanism and prolong the bleeding time.

Guidelines/Precautions

1. Contraindicated in patients with severe bleeding disorders or severe congestive cardiac and renal failure with oliguria or anuria.
2. Use with caution in patients with thrombocytopenia, increased risk of pulmonary edema, or CHF.
3. It is not a substitute for whole blood or plasma because it does not have oxygen-carrying capacity or contain plasma proteins such as coagulation factors.

Principal Adverse Reactions

Cardiovascular: Circulatory overload.
Pulmonary: Pulmonary edema, wheezing.
CNS: Headache.
GI: Vomiting.
Allergic: Urticaria, anaphylactoid reactions.
Other: Mild temperature elevation, muscle pain.

HYDRALAZINE HCL (APRESOLINE)

Use(s): Antihypertensive, treatment of congestive heart failure.
Dosing: IV and IM, 2.5–40 mg (0.1–0.2 mg/kg); PO, 10–100 mg qid; higher doses are required in rapid acetylators.
Elimination: Hepatic (acetylation).
How Supplied: Injection, 20 mg/mL; tablets, 10 mg, 25 mg, 50 mg, and 100 mg.

Pharmacology

This phthalazine derivative lowers blood pressure almost exclusively by a direct relaxant effect on arteriolar smooth muscle. The vasodilation probably reflects hydralazine-related interference with calcium ion transport in vascular smooth muscle. Decrease in blood pressure is accompanied by an increase in heart rate, only partially explained by a reflex increase, and by increases in cardiac output and stroke volume. The drug maintains or increases renal and cerebral blood flow. It also increases plasma renin activity.

Pharmacokinetics

Onset of Action: IV, 5–20 min; IM, 10–30 min; PO, 30–120 min.
Peak Effect: IV, 10–80 min; IM, 20–80 min.
Duration of Action: IV, 2–4 hr; IM/PO, 2–8 hr.
Interaction/Toxicity: Reduced pressor responses to epinephrine; enhanced hypotensive effects in patients receiving diuretics, MAO inhibitors, diazoxide, and other antihypertensives; enhances defluorination of enflurane; lower bioavailability in rapid acetylators (30%) compared with slow acetylators (50%).

Guidelines/Precautions

1. Use cautiously in patients with coronary artery disease, mitral valvular rheumatic heart disease, and patients receiving MAO inhibitors.
2. Systemic lupus erythematosus (SLE) syndrome is dose related and occurs more frequently in patients receiving doses >200 mg/kg for extended periods. Genetically slow acetylators are especially predisposed.

Principal Adverse Reactions

Cardiovascular: Hypotension, paradoxical pressor response, tachycardia, palpitations, angina.
Pulmonary: Dyspnea, nasal congestion.
CNS: Peripheral neuritis, depression, anxiety, headache, dizziness.
GI: Nausea, vomiting, diarrhea.
Dermatologic: SLE-like syndrome.
Allergic: Rash, urticaria, eosinophilia, hypersensitivity.
Hematologic: Leukopenia, splenomegaly, agranulocytosis.

HYDROCORTISONE (HYDROCORTISONE SODIUM SUCCINATE, SOLU-CORTEF, HYDROCORTISONE CYPIONATE, HYDROCORTISONE SODIUM PHOSPHATE, HYDROCORTISONE ACETATE*)

Use(s): Anti-inflammatory, treatment of allergic reactions, steroid replacement, organ transplantation.
Dosing: IV/IM: 20–300 mg (1–2 mg/kg) q2–10h prn.
  Life-threatening shock: IV, 0.5–2 g (50 mg/kg) q2–6h.
  Steroid replacement: IV, 50–100 mg before, during, and after surgery. PO, 5–30 mg bid to qid for severe inflammation and adrenal insufficiency.
  Intraarticular/intratissue: 10–50 mg (repeat at 1–3 wk).
Elimination: Hepatic.
How Supplied: Injection, 20 mg/mL, 25 mg/mL, 50 mg/mL, 125 mg/mL; tablets: 5 mg, 10 mg, 20 mg; oral suspension 10 mg/5 mL.

*Hydrocortisone acetate *not* for IV use.

Pharmacology

A corticosteroid secreted by the adrenal cortex, hydrocortisone has weak antiinflammatory and potent mineralocorticoid activity. It has a rapid onset but short duration of action. It suppresses the hypothalamic-pituitary-adrenal axis.

Pharmacokinetics

Onset of Action: IV/IM, Few minutes.
Peak Effect: IV/IM, <1 hr.
Duration of Action: 8–12 hr (half-life).
Interaction/Toxicity: Clearance enhanced by phenytoin, phenobarbital, ephedrine, and rifampin; altered response to coumarin anticoagulants; enhanced effect in patients with hypothyroidism and cirrhosis; interacts with anticholinesterase agents (e.g., neostigmine) to produce severe weakness in patients with myasthenia gravis; potassium-wasting effects enhanced with potassium-depleting diuretics (e.g., thiazides, furosemide); diminished response to toxoids and live or inactivated vaccines.

Guidelines/Precautions

1. Contraindicated in systemic fungal infections.
2. Use cautiously in patients with ocular herpes simplex for fear of corneal perforation.
3. In patients on corticosteroid therapy subjected to any unusual stress, increase dosage of rapidly acting corticosteroid before, during, and after the stressful situation. Supplemental steroids should be empirically administered to all patients who have received daily steroid replacement for at least 1 wk in the year prior to surgery.
4. Hydrocortisone acetate is not for IV use.

Principal Adverse Reactions

Cardiovascular: Arrhythmias, hypertension, CHF in susceptible patients.
CNS: Seizures, increased intracranial pressure, psychic disturbance.
Fluid and Electrolyte: Sodium retention, fluid retention, hypokalemia.
Musculoskeletal: Weakness, myopathy, osteoporosis.
Endocrine: Growth suppression, secondary adrenocortical and pi-

tuitary unresponsiveness to stress, increased requirement for insulin.
GI: Increased appetite, nausea.
Other: Thromboembolism, weight gain, protein catabolism, glaucoma, increased intraocular tension, erythema, impaired wound healing; diminishes response to toxoids and live or inactivated vaccines; increases susceptibility to and masks symptoms of infection.

HYDROMORPHONE HCL (DILAUDID, DILAUDID HP)*

Use(s): Premedication, analgesia, anesthesia, control of persistent nonproductive cough.
Dosing: Analgesia: Slow IV, 0.5–2 mg; IM/SC, 2–4 mg; PO, 2–4 mg q4–6h prn for pain. Rectal, 3 mg q6–8h. Spinal, 0.1–2.0 mg (2–4 μg/kg). Epidural (bolus), 1–2 mg (20–40 μg/kg) (infusion), 0.15–0.3 mg/hr.
Patient-controlled IV analgesia, (bolus), 0.1–0.5 mg; (infusion), 0.1–0.5 mg/hr; lockout interval, 5–15 min.
Patient-controlled epidural analgesia (bolus), 0.15–0.3 mg; (infusion), 0.15–0.3 mg/hr; lockout interval, 15–30 min.
Antitussive: PO, 0.5–1 mg q3–4h.
Elimination: Hepatic.
How Supplied: Injection: 1 mg/mL, 2 mg/mL, 3 mg/mL, 4 mg/mL; injection: Dilaudid-HP, 10 mg/mL; tablets: 1 mg, 2 mg, 3 mg, 4 mg; rectal suppositories, 3 mg.
Dilution for Infusion: IV, 5 mg in 100 mL NS (50 μg/mL); epidural, 5 mg in 100 mL local anesthetic or (preservative-free) NS solution (50 μg/mL).

Pharmacology

An opiate agonist, which is a hydrogenated ketone of morphine. As an analgesic hydromorphone, it is 7 times more potent than

*For epidural/intrathecal precautions, see Alfentanil, Guidelines/Precautions, items 5 and 6, pp 4–5.

morphine. Primary effects are on the CNS and organs containing smooth muscle. It produces analgesia, drowsiness, euphoria, dose-related depression of respiration, interference with adrenocortical response to stress (at high doses), and reduction in peripheral resistance (arteriolar and venous dilation), with little or no effect on cardiac index. It releases histamine, which can cause pruritus. It may induce nausea and vomiting by activating the chemoreceptor trigger zone. It depresses the cough reflex by a direct effect on the cough centers in the medulla.

Pharmacokinetics

Onset of Action: IV, almost immediate; IM, PO, and SC, 15–30 min; rectal, 10–15 min; epidural, 5 min.
Peak Effect: IV, 5–20 min; IM/PO/SC, 30–60 min; epidural, 30 min.
Duration of Action: IV, 2–4 hr; IM/PO/SC, 4–6 hr; rectal, 6–8 hr; epidural, 10–16 hr.
Interaction/Toxicity: CNS and circulatory depressant effects potentiated by alcohol, sedatives, antihistamines, phenothiazines, butyrophenones, MAO inhibitors, and tricyclic antidepressants; may decrease the effect of diuretics in patients with CHF; analgesia enhanced by α_2-agonists, e.g., clonidine.

Guidelines/Precautions

1. Reduce dose in elderly, hypovolemic, or high-risk surgical patients and with concomitant use of sedatives and other narcotics.
2. The narcotic antagonist naloxone is a specific antidote ($\geq 0.2–0.4$ mg IV). Reversal of narcotic effect may lead to onset of pain and release of catecholamines.
3. Crosses the placental barrier, and usage in labor may produce depression of respiration in the neonate. Resuscitation may be required; have naloxone available.
4. Do not confuse the highly concentrated Dilaudid-HP (10 mg/mL) with other standard parenteral formulations. It is intended for use in narcotic-tolerant patients.

Principal Adverse Reactions

Cardiovascular: Hypotension, hypertension, bradycardia, arrhythmias, chest wall rigidity.

Pulmonary: Bronchospasm, laryngospasm.
CNS: Blurred vision, syncope, euphoria, dysphoria.
GU: Urinary retention, antidiuretic effect, ureteral spasm.
GI: Biliary tract spasm, constipation, anorexia, nausea, vomiting.
Allergic: Pruritus, urticaria.
Musculoskeletal: Chest wall rigidity.

ISOPROTERENOL HCL (ISUPREL, MEDIHALER-ISO)

Use(s): Chronotrope, inotrope, bronchodilator, treatment of bradyarrhythmias, carotid sinus hypersensitivity, heart block; management of shock (hypoperfusion) syndromes; resuscitation in cardiac arrest.

Dosing: Arrhythmias/resuscitation: IM/SC, 0.2 mg; IV push, 0.02–0.06 mg; infusion, 2–20 μg/min (0.02–0.15 μg/kg/min) (rates >30 μg/min have been used in advanced stages of shock); sublingual: 10 mg, then 5–50 mg prn.

Bronchospasm: Metered dose inhaler: 120–262 μg (1–2 inhalations of 0.25% solution) q3–4h; do not take >2 inhalations at any 1 time. Maximum, 6 inhalations/hr. Nebulizer: Adults, 1:200 solution, dilute 0.5 mL in 2.5 mL NS solution (deliver solution over 10–20 min), give treatment q4h; Children, 1:200 solution (dilute 0.25 ml in 2.5 mL NS solution).

Elimination: Hepatic.

How Supplied: Injection: 1:50,000 solution (0.02 mg/mL); 1:5000 solution (0.2 mg/mL).
Glossets: Sublingual/rectal, 10 mg, 15 mg.
Aerosol: 80 μg, 120 μg, 131 μg, 160 μg/metered spray.
Solution for nebulization: 0.031%, 0.062%, 0.25%, 0.5%, 1%.

Dilution for Infusion: 3 mg in 250 mL D_5W or NS solution (12 μg/mL).

Pharmacology

A synthetic sympathomimetic amine that is structurally related to epinephrine but acts almost exclusively on β_1- and β_2-adrenergic receptors such as those in heart, bronchiolar smooth muscle, skeletal muscle vasculature, and alimentary tract. It produces a positive inotropic and chronotropic effect and increases the rate of discharge of cardiac pacemakers. Isoproterenol decreases systemic and pulmonary vascular resistance and increases coronary and renal blood flow. It has potent relaxing effects on bronchiolar smooth muscle.

Pharmacokinetics

Onset of Action: IV, immediate; inhalation, 2–5 min; sublingual/SC, 15–30 min.
Peak Effect: IV, 1 min.
Duration of Action: IV, 1–5 min; inhalation, 30 min–2 hr; sublingual/SC, 1–2 hr.
Interaction/Toxicity: Arrhythmias with concomitant use of volatile anesthetics and other sympathomimetics such as epinephrine; effects antagonized by β-adrenergic-blocking drugs such as propranolol.

Guidelines/Precautions

1. Contraindicated in patients with tachyarrhythmias, tachycardia, heart block caused by digitalis intoxication; not a substitute for the replacement of blood, plasma, fluids, and electrolytes.
2. May exacerbate ischemia and/or hypertension when used for chronotropic support; electronic pacing provides better control.
3. Paradoxical bronchoconstriction has occasionally occurred with repeated; excessive inhalational use.

Principal Adverse Reactions

Cardiovascular: Tachyarrhythmias, palpitation, angina, paradoxical precipitation of Adams-Stokes attacks.
Pulmonary: Pulmonary edema.
CNS: Headache, dizziness, tremors.
GI: Nausea, vomiting, anorexia.

KETAMINE HCL (KETALAR)*

Use(s): Dissociative anesthetic; induction and maintenance of anesthesia, especially in hypovolemic or high-risk patients; sole anesthetic for short surgical procedures.

Dosing: Sedation and analgesia: IV, 0.5–1 mg/kg.

IM, 2.5–5 mg/kg. PO, 5–6 mg/kg. Dilute injectate solution in 5–10 mL (0.2 mL/kg) cola-flavored drink.

Induction: IV, 1–2.5 mg/kg; IM/rectal, 5–10 mg/kg.

Infusion: 15–80 μg/kg/min (augment with 2–5 mg IV diazepam or 1–2 mg IV midazolam as needed). Epidural/caudal: 0.5 mg/kg. Dilute in NS or local anesthetic (1 mL/kg).

Elimination: Hepatic.

How Supplied: Injection: 10 mg/mL, 50 mg/mL, 100 mg/mL.

Dilution for Infusion: 250 mg in 250 mL D_5W or NS solution (1 mg/mL).

Pharmacology

This phencyclidine derivative produces rapid-acting dissociative anesthesia characterized by normal or slightly enhanced laryngeal reflexes, normal or slightly enhanced skeletal muscle tone, respiratory stimulation, and occasionally a transient and minimal respiratory depression. The central sympathetic stimulation, neuronal release, of catecholamines and inhibition of neuronal uptake of catecholamines usually overrides the direct myocardial depressant effects of ketamine. Hemodynamic effects (that depend on intact sympathetic responses) include increases in systemic and pulmonary arterial pressure, heart rate, and cardiac output. Ketamine is a useful anesthetic agent in patients with hemodynamic compromise based on either hypovolemia or intrinsic cardiac (but not coronary artery) disease, e.g., cardiac tamponade. It is a bronchial smooth muscle relaxant and is as effective as the inhalational anesthetics in preventing experimentally induced bronchospasm. Cerebral blood flow and intracranial pressure are increased in the presence of normocapnia. Ketamine increases salivary and tracheobroncheal secretions. It does not release histamine.

*For epidural/intrathecal precautions, see Alfentanil, Guidelines.Precautions, item 5 and 6, pp. 4–5.

Pharmacokinetics

Onset of Action: IV, within 30 sec; IM/rectal, 3–4 min.
Peak Effect: IV, 1 min.
Duration of Action: IV, 5–15 min; IM/rectal, 12–25 min.
Interaction/Toxicity: Emergence delirium; decreased requirements for volatile anesthetics; hemodynamic depression may occur in the presence of α-blockers, β-blockers calcium channel blockers, benzodiazepines, opioids, and inhalational anesthetics; enhancement of depolarizing and nondepolarizing neuromuscular blockers; reduction of seizure threshold when administered with aminophylline.

Guidelines/Precautions

1. Critically ill patients with catecholamine depletion may respond to ketamine with unexpected reductions in blood pressure and cardiac output.
2. Emergence reactions (dreaming, hallucinations, confusion) are more common in adults (15 to 65 years), with high doses, and with rapid administration, and are reduced by premedication with benzodiazepines and droperidol.
3. Do not mix with barbiturates in same syringe. Precipitate formation occurs.
4. Use with caution in patients with severe hypertension ischemic heart disease, those with increased intracranial pressure, chronic alcoholics, and the acutely alcohol-intoxicated patient.
5. Increased salivary secretions may cause upper airway obstruction and laryngospasm especially in children. Administer an antisialagogue, e.g., glycopyrrolate, preoperatively.
6. Avoid IM ketamine sedation (1–2 mg/kg) in preterm infants. It may cause prolonged apnea with bradycardia.

Principal Adverse Reactions

Cardiovascular: Hypertension, tachycardia, hypotension, arrhythmias bradycardia.
Pulmonary: Respiratory depression, apnea, laryngospasm.
CNS: Tonic, clonic movements, emergence delirium.
GI: Hypersalivation, nausea, vomiting.
Eye: Diplopia, nystagmus, slight elevation in intraocular tension.

KETOROLAC TROMETHAMINE (TORADOL)

Use(s): Analgesia.
Dosing: Loading IM, 30–60 mg; maintenance IM, 15–30 mg q6h and/or 10 mg PO q4–6h prn; maximum total dose, 150 mg for the first day and 120 mg/day thereafter. IV route has not been approved for general clinical use in the United States.
Elimination: Hepatic, renal.
How Supplied: Injection: IM, 15 mg/mL, 30 mg/mL.
Tablets: 10 mg.

Pharmacology

This NSAID exhibits analgesic, anti-inflammatory, and antipyretic activity. It inhibits synthesis of prostaglandins and may be considered a peripherally acting analgesic. Analgesic potency of 30 mg ketorolac is equivalent to 9 mg morphine, with less drowsiness, nausea, and vomiting, and no significant change in ventilatory function. It inhibits platelet aggregation and prolongs bleeding time. Inhibition of platelet function disappears within 24–48 hr after the drug is discontinued. It does not affect platelet count, PT, or partial thromboplastin time (PTT).

Pharmacokinetics

Onset of Action: IM, <10 min; PO, 1 hr.
Peak Effect: IM/PO, 1–3 hr.
Duration of Action: IM/PO, 3–7 hr.
Interaction/Toxicity: Effects potentiated by concomitant use of salicylates; enhances toxicity of lithium, methotrexate; may precipitate renal failure in patients with impaired renal function, heart failure, and liver dysfunction, patients on diuretic therapy, and the elderly.

Guidelines/Precautions

1. Use with caution in patients with impaired renal or hepatic function. It may cause fluid retention and edema in patients with cardiac decompensation or hypertension.
2. Observe carefully patients with coagulation disorders and those receiving drug therapy that interferes with hemostasis.
3. Contraindicated in patients with previously demonstrated hypersensitivity to ketorolac or with the complete or partial syn-

drome of nasal polyps, angioedema, or bronchospastic reactivity to aspirin or other NSAIDs.
4. Do not use for obstetric analgesia; not recommended for premedication because it prolongs bleeding time.

Principal Adverse Reactions

Cardiovascular: Vasodilation, pallor, angina.
Pulmonary: Dyspnea, asthma.
CNS: Drowsiness, dizziness, headache, sweating, depression, euphoria.
GI: Ulceration, bleeding, dyspepsia, nausea, vomiting, diarrhea, GI pain.
Dermatologic: Pruritus, urticaria.

LABETALOL HCL (NORMODYNE, TRANDATE)

Use(s): Antihypertensive.
Dosing: IV bolus, 2.5–20 mg (0.25 mg/kg) slowly over 2 min (titrate to blood pressure response).
 Infusion, 0.5–2 mg/min. Maximum cumulative dose of 1–4 mg/kg; PO, 100–400 mg bid.
Elimination: Hepatic; urine and feces.
How Supplied: Injection, 5 mg/mL; tablets, 100 mg, 200 mg, 300 mg.
Dilution for Iufusion: 200 mg in 200 mL D_5W or NS (1 mg/mL).

Pharmacology

An adrenergic receptor–blocking agent with mild α_1- and predominant β-adrenergic receptor–blocking actions. Produces dose-related decrease in blood pressure without reflex tachycardia and without profound reduction in heart rate. β_2-Adrenergic blockade may result in bronchoconstriction in patients subject to bronchospasm.

Pharmacokinetics

Onset of Action: IV, 2–5 min; PO, 20 min–2 hr.
Peak Effect: IV, 5–15 min; PO, 1–4 hr.
Duration of Action: IV, 2–4 hr; PO, 8–24 hr.
Interaction/Toxicity: Bioavailability increased by cimetidine; increased resistance to β-agonist bronchodilators, blunts reflex

tachycardia produced by nitroglycerin; hypotensive effect potentiated by volatile anesthetics.

Guidelines/Precautions

1. Contraindicated in bronchial asthma, overt cardiac failure, greater than first-degree heart block, cardiogenic shock, and severe bradycardia.
2. Manifestations of excessive vagal tone and myocardial depression (profound bradycardia, hypotension) may be corrected with IV atropine (1–2 mg), IV isoproterenol (0.02–0.15 μg/kg/min), IV glucagon (1–5 mg), transvenous cardiac pacemaker, or a vasopressor (e.g., epinephrine, dopamine, dobutamine).
3. Increased risk of ischemia or infarction in patients with coronary artery disease if drug is withdrawn abruptly.
4. May block signs of acute hypoglycemia.

Principal Adverse Reactions

Cardiovascular: Hypotension, bradycardia, ventricular arrhythmias, CHF, chest pain.
Pulmonary: Dyspnea, bronchospasm.
CNS: Headache, drowsiness, paresthesia, vertigo, tremor, mental depression, fatigue, numbness.
GI: Diarrhea, cholestasis, elevated liver enzyme levels.
Dermatologic: Rashes.
Other: SLE, positive antinuclear antibody (ANA) titer.

LIDOCAINE HCL (XYLOCAINE)*

Use(s): Regional anesthesia; treatment of ventricular arrhythmias, especially when associated with acute myocardial infarction or cardiac surgery, attenuation of pressor response to intubation.
Dosing: Antiarrhythmic: Slow IV bolus, 1 mg/kg (1%–2% solution) followed by 0.5 mg/kg every 2–5 min (to maximum of 3 mg/kg/hr). Infusion (0.1% solution), 1–4 mg/min (20–50 μg/kg/min). IM, 4–5 mg/kg; may be

---

*For additional precautions, see Bupivacaine, Guidelines/Precautions, items 8 to 10, p 20.

repeated 60–90 min later. Reduce doses in the elderly, patients with heart failure or liver disease, or those who are receiving β-blockers or cimetidine.

Local anesthesia: Topical, 0.6–3 mg/kg (2%–4% solution). Infiltration/peripheral nerve block, 0.5–5 mg/kg (0.5%–2% solution). Transtracheal, 80–120 mg (2–3 mL of 4% solution). Superior laryngeal nerve, 40–60 mg (2–3 mL of 2% solution on each side). Stellate ganglion, 50 mg (5 mL of 1% solution).

IV regional: Upper extremities, 200–250 mg (40–50 mL of 0.5% solution). Lower extremities, 250–300 mg (100–120 mL of 0.25% solution). Do not add epinephrine for IV regional block.

Brachial plexus block: 300–400 mg (30–40 mL of 1% solution). Children, 0.2–0.33 mL/kg.

Caudal: 150–300 mg (15–20 mL of 1% or 1.5% solution). Children, 0.4–0.7 mL/kg (L2–T10 level of anesthesia).

Epidural: (bolus), 200–400 mg (1%–2% solution). Children, 7–9 mg/kg. (Infusion) 8–12 mL/hr (0.5% solution). Children, 0.2–0.35 mL/kg/hr. Rate of onset and potency of local anesthetic action may be enhanced by carbonation. (Add 1 mL 8.4% sodium bicarbonate with 10 mL of 0.5%–2% lidocaine. Do not use if there is precipitation).

Spinal bolus/infusion: 50–100 mg (5% solution with glucose 7.5%). Therapeutic level, 1.5–6 μg/mL. Maximum safe dose, 4 mg/kg without epinephrine, 7 mg/kg with epinephrine 1:200,000.

Doses for epidural or spinal anesthesia should be reduced in pregnant patients. Solutions containing preservatives should not be used for spinal, epidural, or caudal block. IV: use only lidocaine injection without preservatives clearly labeled for IV use.

Elimination: Hepatic, pulmonary.

How Supplied: Parenteral administration: injection for IM injection, 10%; injection for direct IV, 1%, 2%; injection for IV admixture, 4%, 10%, 20%; injection for IV infusion, 0.2%, 0.4%, 0.8%.

Infiltration/peripheral nerve block: 0.5%, 1%, 1.5%, 2% with or without epinephrine, 1:50,000, 1:100,000, 1:200,000.

Epidural: 1%, 1.5%, 2% preservative free.
Spinal (hyperbaric solution): 1.5%, 5% solution with 7.5% dextrose/glucose.
Laryngotracheal: with laryngotracheal cannula, 4% sterile solution.
Dilution for Infusion: IV, 2 g in 500 mL D_5W (4 mg/mL); epidural, 20 mL 1% in 20 mL (preservative-free) NS (0.5%) solution.

Pharmacology

This amide-derivative local anesthetic has a rapid onset of action. It stabilizes neuronal membrane by inhibiting the sodium flux required for the initiation and conduction of impulses. The drug is also a class 1B antiarrhythmic agent, which suppresses automaticity and shortens the effective refractory period and action potential duration of the His-Purkinje system. Action potential duration and effective refractory period of ventricular muscle are also decreased. Therapeutic doses do not significantly decrease systemic arterial blood pressure, myocardial contractility, or cardiac output. Repeated doses cause significant increases in blood level because of slow accumulation.

Pharmacokinetics

Onset: IV (antiarrhythmic effects), 45–90 sec; infiltration, 0.5–1 min; epidural, 5–15 min.
Peak Effect: IV (antiarrhythmic effects), 1–2 min; infiltration and epidural, <30 min.
Duration: IV (antiarrhythmic effects), 10–20 min; infiltration, 0.5–1 hr; with epinephrine, 2–6 hr; epidural, 1–3 hr (prolonged with epinephrine).
Interaction/Toxicity: Cardiac effects with other antiarrhythmics such as phenytoin, procainamide, propranolol, or quinidine may be additive or antagonistic, may potentiate the neuromuscular blocking effect of succinylcholine, tubocurarine; reduced clearance with concomitant use of β-blocking agents, cimetidine; seizures, respiratory, and circulatory depression at high plasma levels; benzodiazepines increase seizure threshold; duration of local or regional anesthesia prolonged by vasoconstrictor agents, e.g., epinephrine.

Guidelines/Precautions

1. Use with caution in patients with hypovolemia, severe CHF, shock, and all forms of heart block.
2. Contraindicated in patients with hypersensitivity to amide-type local anesthetics.
3. Benzodiazepines increase seizure threshold.
4. Use for paracervical block associated with fetal bradycardia and acidosis.
5. In IV regional blocks, deflate the cuff after 40 min and not less than 20 min. Between 20 and 40 min the cuff can be deflated, reinflated immediately, and finally deflated after 1 min to reduce the sudden absorption of anesthetic into the systemic circulation.
6. Cauda equina syndrome with permanent neurologic deficit has occurred in patients receiving >100 mg of a 5% lidocaine solution with a continuous spinal technique.

Principal Adverse Reactions

Cardiovascular: Hypotension, bradycardia, arrhythmias, heart block.
Pulmonary: Respiratory depression, arrest.
CNS: Tinnitus, seizures, loss of hearing, euphoria, anxiety, diplopia, postspinal headache, arachnoiditis, palsies.
Allergic: Urticaria, pruritus, angioneurotic edema.
Epidural/Caudal/Spinal: High spinal, loss of bladder and bowel control, permanent motor, sensory, autonomic (sphincter control), deficit of lower segments.

LORAZEPAM (ATIVAN)

Use(s): Premedication, amnesia, induction agent, treatment of acute alcohol withdrawal, and chemotherapy induced nausea and vomiting.
Dosing: Sedation: IV/deep IM, 1–2 mg (0.04 mg/kg) (maximum dose, 4 mg); dilute with equal volume D_5W or NS solution); PO, 2 mg bid or tid (elderly: 1–2 mg/day in divided doses).
Induction: IV, 0.5–1 mg/kg.

Elimination: Hepatic, renal.
How Supplied: Injection, 2 mg/mL, 4 mg/mL; tablets, 0.5 mg, 1 mg, 2 mg.

Pharmacology

This benzodiazepine produces a dose-related sedation, relief of preoperative anxiety, and lack of recall of events relating to the day of surgery in a majority of patients. Like other benzodiazepines, the drug is thought to influence the effect of GABA, an inhibitory neurotransmitter, in the brain. It produces minimal depressant effects on ventilation and circulation in the absence of other CNS depressant drugs. Unpredictable blood level–CNS response relationship. It is intermediate in speed of onset compared with other benzodiazepines.

Pharmacokinetics

Onset of Action: IV, 1–5 min; IM, 15–30 min; PO, 1–6 hr.
Peak Effect: IV, 15–20 min; PO, 2 hr.
Duration of Action: IV/IM/PO, 6–24 hr.
Interaction/Toxicity: CNS and circulatory depressant effects potentiated by cimetidine, alcohol, narcotics, sedatives, barbiturates, phenothiazines, MAO inhibitors, and volatile anesthetics; decreased requirements for volatile anesthetics; effects antagonized by flumazenil.

Guidelines/Precautions

1. Intra-arterial injection may produce arteriospasm resulting in gangrene. Treat with local infiltration of phentolamine (5–10 mg in 10 mL NS) and, if necessary, sympathetic block.
2. For optimal amnesic effects, administer IV 15–20 min or PO 2 hr before anticipated operative procedure.
3. Unexpected hypotension and respiratory depression may occur when combined with opioids.
4. Use with caution in elderly patients and patients with limited pulmonary reserve because excessive sedation and hypoventilation may occur.
5. Not for use in children <12 yr old.
6. Treat overdose with supportive measures and flumazenil (slow IV, 0.2–1 mg).
7. Contraindicated in patients with known hypersensitivity to

benzodiazepines or any ingredients in the parenteral formulation (i.e., polyethylene glycol, propylene glycol, or benzyl alcohol) and in patients with acute angle-closure glaucoma.

Principal Adverse Reactions

Cardiovascular: Hypotension, hypertension, bradycardia, tachycardia.
Pulmonary: Respiratory depression.
CNS: Sedation, dizziness, weakness, depression, agitation, amnesia.
Psychologic: Hysteria, psychosis.
GI: Change in appetite.
Other: Visual disturbances, urticaria, pruritus.

MAGNESIUM SULFATE (MAGNESIUM SULFATE)

Use(s): Prevention and control of seizures in toxemia/eclampsia of pregnancy, epilepsy, nephritis and hypomagnesemia; treatment of acute magnesium deficiency; tocolytic therapy; adjunctive therapy of acute MI, *torsades de pointes* ventricular tachycardia, and hypokalemia-related arrhythmias.
Dosing: Toxemia: Slow IV, 1–4 g 10%–20% solution then infusion, 1–2 g/hr; IM, 1–5 g 25%–50% solution q4h prn (use 25% dilution for children); therapeutic plasma level, 4–6 mEq/L.

Hypomagnesemia: IV, 10–15 mg/kg 10%–20% solution over 15–20 min then infusion, 1 g/hr; IM, 10–15 mg/kg q6h for 4 doses; PO, 3 g q6h for 4 doses (normal plasma level, 1.5–2.2 mEq/L).

Elimination: Renal.
How Supplied: Injection: 10% (0.8 mEq/100 mg/mL), 12.5% (1 mEq/125 mg/mL), 50% (4 mEq/500 mg/mL).
Dilution for Infusion: 10 g in 1000 ml D_5W (10 mg/mL).

Pharmacology

This mineral is present in the body and distributed principally in intracellular space. It regulates presynaptic release of acetylcholine from nerve endings, activates enzyme systems such as alkaline phosphatase, and is an essential cofactor in oxidative phosphorylation. At the neuromuscular junction, it decreases acetylcholine release, reduces the sensitivity of the motor end plate to acetylcholine, and decreases the amplitude of the motor end plate potential. These effects are opposed by calcium. Hypocalcemia and hypokalemia often follow low serum levels of magnesium. Magnesium exerts CNS and respiratory depressant effects. It slows the rate of sinoatrial node impulse formation and prolongs conduction time. The drug produces vasodilation and high doses decrease arterial pressure.

Pharmacokinetics

Onset of Action: IV, immediate; IM, <1 hr.
Peak Effect: IV, few minutes; IM, 1–3 hr.
Duration of Action: IV, 30 min; IM, 3–4 hr.
Interaction/Toxicity: Potentiates both depolarizing and nondepolarizing muscle relaxants; cardiac depression, respiratory paralysis, loss of deep tendon reflexes at serum levels >10–12 mEq/L; potentiates CNS depressant effects of sedatives, narcotics, volatile anesthetics; CNS depression and peripheral neuromuscular blockade provided by hypermagnesemia antagonized by calcium.

Guidelines/Precautions

1. Treat life-threatening hypermagnesemia with 5–10 mEq calcium IV (10–20 ml 10% calcium gluconate), followed by fluid loading and drug-induced diuresis.
2. Periodic monitoring of plasma magnesium concentrations is essential during magnesium therapy. Disappearance of the patellar reflex is a useful clinical sign to detect the onset of magnesium intoxication. Knee jerk reflex should be tested before repeat doses, and if they are absent, no additional magnesium should be given until they return.
3. Contraindicated in heart block or in patients with extensive myocardial damage.
4. Maintain urine output at a minimum of 100 mL q4h.

Principal Adverse Reactions

Cardiovascular: Hypotension, circulatory collapse, heart block.
Pulmonary: Respiratory paralysis.
CNS: Flaccid paralysis, depressed reflexes.
Metabolic: Hypocalcemia.
Other: Flushing, sweating, hypothermia.

MANNITOL (OSMITROL)

Use(s): Diuretic, differential diagnosis of acute oliguria, "renal protection" in presence of myoglobin, hemoglobinuria, and for aortic aneurysmectomy; treatment of increased intracranial and intraocular pressure.

Dosing: Acute oliguria: Infusion, 0.25–1 g/kg (5%–25% solution).

Reduction of intracranial and intraocular pressure: Infusion, 1.5–2 g/kg (6–8 mL/kg 20%–25% solution).

Elimination: Renal.

How Supplied: 5%, 10%, 15%, 20%, 25% solution.

Pharmacology

A six-carbon sugar that is pharmacologically inert and resists metabolism. Because it is freely filtered at the glomerulus, mannitol raises the osmolarity of the renal tubular fluid and inhibits tubular reabsorption of water and electrolytes. Urinary excretion of water, sodium, chloride, and bicarbonate ions are increased. Urinary pH is not altered. Plasma osmolarity is also increased with an acute expansion of intravascular fluid volume. Shift of fluid from extracellular to intracellular sites decreases brain size and may increase renal blood flow.

Pharmacokinetics

Onset of Action: Diuresis, 15–60 min.; reduction of intraocular pressure, 30–60 min; intracranial pressure, <15 min.

Peak Effect: Diuresis, 1 hr; reduction of intraocular pressure, 1–2 hr.

Duration of Action: Diuresis, 3–8 hr. reduction of intraocular pressure, 4–6 hr; intraocular pressure, 3–8 hr.

Interaction/Toxicity: Increases urinary excretion of lithium.

Guidelines/Precautions

1. If urine output continues to decline during infusion, review the patient's clinical status and suspend infusion if necessary. Accumulation of mannitol may result in overexpansion of the extracellular fluid, which may intensify existing or latent CHF and pulmonary edema.
2. Periodically monitor fluid and electrolyte values.

3. If blood-brain barrier is not intact, mannitol may enter the brain, producing rebound cerebral edema.
4. Contraindicated in severe pulmonary congestion, frank pulmonary edema, or anuria caused by severe renal disease. May be contraindicated with intracerebral bleeding, aneurysm, or arteriovenous malformation, because by shrinking healthy brain tissue, hematoma may expand and fragile bridging veins may rupture, producing subdural hematoma.
5. Do not give electrolyte-free mannitol solutions with blood. If blood is given simultaneously, add at least 20 mEq sodium chloride to each liter of mannitol solution to avoid pseudoagglutination.
6. Obligatory response after rapid infusion may further aggravate preexisting hemoconcentration.

Principal Adverse Reactions

Cardiovascular: Edema, hypertension, hypotension, tachycardia, chest pain.
Pulmonary: Pulmonary edema.
CNS: Seizures, headaches, blurred vision, dizziness.
GI: Nausea, vomiting, diarrhea.
Dermatologic: Skin necrosis, urticaria.
Metabolic: Hypernatremia, hyponatremia, hyperkalemia, acidosis, dehydration.
Other: Chills, fever, thirst, dry mouth, rhinitis.

MEPERIDINE HCL (DEMEROL)*

Use(s): Premedication, analgesia.
Dosing: IV/IM/PO: 25–75 mg (0.5–2 mg/kg).
　　　　　Epidural: Bolus, 1–2 mg/kg; infusion, 10–20 mg/hr.
　　　　　Spinal: Bolus, 0.2–1 mg/kg infusion, 5–10 mg/hr.
　　　　　Patient-controlled analgesia: IV/epidural (bolus), 5–30 mg; (infusion), 5–10 mg/hr; lockout interval: 5–15 min.
Elimination: Hepatic.

*For epidural/intrathecal precautions, see Alfentanil, Guidelines/Precautions, items 5 and 6, pp 4–5.

How Supplied: Injection: 10 mg/mL, 25 mg/mL, 50 mg/mL, 75 mg/mL, 100 mg/mL; tablets: 50 mg, 100 mg; oral solution: 50 mg/5 mL.

Dilution for Infusion: IV, 100 mg in 50 mL D_5W or NS (2 mg/mL) epidural, 100 mg in 50 mL local anesthetic or (preservative-free) NS solution (2 mg/mL).

Pharmacology

This synthetic opioid agonist is approximately one tenth as potent as morphine, with a slightly more rapid onset and shorter duration of action. Meperidine has mild vagolytic and antispasmodic effects. It may produce orthostatic hypotension at therapeutic doses and has a direct myocardial depressant effect at high doses.

Pharmacokinetics

Onset: PO, 10–45 min; IV, <1 min; IM, 1–5 min; epidural/spinal, 2–12 min.

Peak Effect: PO, <1 hr; IV, 5–20 min; IM, 30–50 min.

Duration of Action: PO/IV/IM, 2–4 hr; epidural spinal, 0.5–3 hr.

Interaction/Toxicity: Cerebral irritation and seizures in large doses; potentiates CNS and cardiovascular depression of narcotics, sedative-hypnotics, volatile anesthetics, tricyclic antidepressants; severe, sometimes fatal, reaction (hyperthermia, hypertension, seizures) with MAO inhibitors; analgesia enhanced by α_2-agonists, e.g., clonidine; aggravates adverse effects of isoniazid; chemically incompatible mixture with barbiturates.

Guidelines/Precautions

1. Severe and occasionally fatal reactions in patients who are receiving or have just received MAO inhibitors. Treat with hydrocortisone IV. Use chlorpromazine IV to treat the associated hypertension.
2. Do not use in high doses for anesthesia.
3. Use with caution in patients with asthma, chronic obstructive pulmonary disease, increased intracranial pressure, supraventricular tachycardia.
4. Reduce doses in elderly, hypovolemic, high-risk surgical patients and with concomitant use of sedatives and other narcotics.

5. Narcotic effects reversed by naloxone ($\geq 0.2 - 0.4$ mg IV). Duration of reversal may be shorter than duration of narcotic effect.
6. Crosses the placental barrier and usage in labor may produce depression of respiration in the neonate. Resuscitation may be required; have naloxone available.

Principal Adverse Reactions

Cardiovascular: Hypotension, cardiac arrest.
Pulmonary: Respiratory depression, arrest, laryngospasm.
CNS: Euphoria, dysphoria, sedation, seizures, psychic dependence.
GI: Constipation, biliary tract spasm.
Musculoskeletal: Chest wall rigidity.
Allergic: Urticaria, pruritus.

MEPHENTERMINE SULFATE (WYAMINE)

Use(s): Inotropic agent, vasoconstrictor.
Dosing: IV/IM, 15–45 mg (0.4 mg/kg); infusion, 0.2–5 mg/min (4–100 µg/kg/min).
Elimination: Hepatic.
How Supplied: Injection, 15 mg/mL, 30 mg/mL.
Dilution for Infusion: 250 mg in 250 mL D_5W (1 mg/mL).

Pharmacology

A synthetic noncatecholamine sympathomimetic that stimulates α- and β-receptors. It acts directly and indirectly by releasing norepinephrine from neuronal storage sites. Mephentermine increases blood pressure, heart rate, and cardiac output primarily by an increase in myocardial contractility and to a lesser degree an increase in peripheral vascular resistance. It increases cerebral blood flow and produces CNS stimulation.

Pharmacokinetics

Onset of Action: IV, 1–5 min; IM, 5–15 min.
Peak Effect: IV, 5 min; IM, 15–60 min.
Duration of Action: IV 15–30 min; IM, 1–2 hr.

Interaction/Toxicity: Increased risk of arrhythmias with use of volatile anesthetics, especially halothane; pressor effect potentiated in patients treated with MAO inhibitors, tricyclic antidepressants, oxytocics; ineffective in patients treated with reserpine or guanethidine; potentiates rather than corrects hypotension secondary to the adrenolytic effects of chlorpromazine.

Guidelines/Precautions

1. Use is not a substitute for the replacement of blood, plasma, fluids, and electrolytes, which should be restored promptly when loss has occurred.
2. Use with caution in patients with severe hypertension or hyperthyroidism.
3. May increase uterine contractions, especially during the third trimester of pregnancy. It is not recommended for use in pregnant women.

Principal Adverse Reactions

Cardiovascular: Hypertension, arrhythmias.
CNS: Anxiety, seizures, euphoria, paranoid psychosis.

MEPIVACAINE HCL (CARBOCAINE, POLOCAINE)*

Use(s): Regional anesthesia.
Dosing: Infiltration, 50–400 mg (0.5%–1.5% solution).
　　　　　Brachial plexus block, 300–400 mg (30–40 mL of 1% solution. Children, 0.2–0.33 mL/kg.
　　　　　Epidural, 150–400 mg (15–20 mL 1%–2% solution); rate of onset and potency of local anesthetic action may be enhanced by carbonation (add 1 mL 8.4% sodium bicarbonate with 10 mL 1%–3% mepivacaine; do not use if there is precipitation)
　　　　　Caudal, 150–400 mg (15–20 mL 1%–2% solution. Children, 0.4–0.7 mL/kg (L2–T10 level of anesthesia).

*For additional precautions, see Bupivacaine, Guidelines/Precautions, items 8 to 10, p 20.

Maximum safe dose, 4 mg/kg without epinephrine, 7 mg/kg with epinephrine 1:200,000.

Solutions containing preservatives should not be used for epidural or caudal block.

Elimination: Hepatic.

How Supplied: Injection, 1%, 1.5%, 2%, 3%.

Pharmacology

This tertiary amine local anesthetic stabilizes the neuronal membrane and prevents the initiation and transmission of impulses. The amide structure is not detoxified by plasma esterases, and metabolism occurs primarily by hepatic microsomal enzymes. Similar to lidocaine in potency and speed of onset, mepivacaine has a slightly longer duration of action and lacks vasodilator activity.

Pharmacokinetics

Onset of Action: Infiltration, 3–5 min; epidural, 5–15 min.
Peak Effect: Infiltration/epidural, 15–45 min.
Duration of Action: Infiltration, 0.75–1.5 hr; with epinephrine, 2–6 hr; epidural, 3–5 hr; prolonged with epinephrine.
Interaction/Toxicity: Reduced clearance with coadministration of β-blockers, cimetidine; seizures, respiratory and circulatory depression at high plasma levels; benzodiazepines increase seizure threshold.

Guidelines/Precaution

1. Do not use for spinal anesthesia.
2. Not recommended for obstetric anesthesia. High neonatal blood levels are due to placental transfer and impaired elimination.
3. Use for paracervical block associated with fetal bradycardia and acidosis.
4. Use with caution in patients with severe disturbance of cardiac rhythm and heart block.
5. Contraindicated in patients with hypersensitivity to amide-type local anesthetics.

Principal Adverse Reactions

Cardiovascular: Hypotension, bradycardia, cardiac arrest.
Pulmonary: Respiratory depression, arrest.

CNS: Tinnitus, seizures, loss of hearing, euphoria, dysphoria.
Allergic: Urticaria, pruritus, angioneurotic edema.
Epidural/Caudal: High spinal, loss of bladder and bowel control, permanent motor, sensory, autonomic (sphincter control) deficit of lower segments.

METHADONE HCL (DOLOPHINE)*

Use(s): Premedication, analgesia, detoxification treatment of narcotic addiction.
Dosing: Analgesia: IV/IM/PO, 2.5–10 mg (0.1 mg/kg) q3–4h.
      Epidural bolus, 1–5 mg (20–100 µg/kg).
      Narcotic abstinence syndrome: PO, 15–120 mg/day (highly individualized).
      Patient-controlled analgesia: IV (bolus), 0.5–3.0 mg; lockout interval, 10–20 min.
Maintenance methadone therapy (>3 wk) may occur only at approved methadone programs.
Elimination: Hepatic.
How Supplied: Injection, 10 mg/mL; tablets, 5 mg, 10 mg, 40 mg; oral solution, 1 mg/mL, 2 mg/mL, and 10 mg/mL.

Pharmacology

A synthetic narcotic analgesic with multiple actions quantitatively similar to those of morphine mainly involving the CNS and organs composed of smooth muscle. The methadone abstinence syndrome, although qualitatively similar to that of morphine, differs in that the onset is slower, the course is more prolonged, and the symptoms are less severe. Cumulative effect occurs with repeated use, resulting in a prolonged duration of action. Oral methadone is approximately half as potent as parenteral.

Pharmacokinetics

Onset of Action: IV, several minutes; IM, 30–60 min; PO, 30–60 min. Epidural, 5–10 min.
Peak Effect: IV, several minutes; IM/PO, 0.5–1 hr.

*For epidural/intrathecal precautions, see Alfentanil, Guidelines/Precautions, items 5 and 6, pp 4–5.

Duration of Action: IV/IM/PO, 4–6 hr. Epidural, 6–10 hr.
Interaction/Toxicity: Blood concentration may be reduced by rifampin, with production of withdrawal symptoms; severe reaction with MAO inhibitors; withdrawal symptoms precipitated by pentazocine in heroin addicts on methadone therapy; potentiates CNS and cardiovascular depressant effects of other narcotic analgesics, volatile anesthetics, phenothiazines, sedative-hypnotics, alcohol, tricyclic antidepressants, analgesia enhanced by α_2-agonists, e.g., clonidine.

Guidelines/Precautions

1. Do not give pentazocine to heroin addicts on methadone.
2. Ineffective for relief of general anxiety.
3. Use with caution in patients with asthma, chronic obstructive pulmonary disease, increased intracranial pressure.
4. Reduce dosage in elderly, hypovolemic, high-risk surgical patients or with use of narcotics and sedative hypnotics.
5. Can produce drug dependence of morphine type and therefore has the potential for being abused.
6. Use of doses >120 mg require special federal approval.
7. Not recommended for obstetric analgesia.

Principal Adverse Reactions

Cardiovascular: Hypotension, circulatory depression, bradycardia, syncope.
Pulmonary: Respiratory depression.
CNS: Euphoria, dysphoria, disorientation.
GU: Urinary retention.
GI: Biliary tract spasm, constipation, anorexia.
Allergic: Rash, pruritus, urticaria.

METHOHEXITAL SODIUM (BREVITAL)

Use(s): Induction agent, supplementation of anesthesia, sole anesthetic for pain-free procedures (e.g., cardioversion).
Dosing: Sedation: IV, 0.25–1 mg/kg.
Induction: IV, 1.5–2.5 mg/kg. IM, 7–10 mg/kg. Rectal, 20–30 mg/kg; 5% aqueous solution for children

(500 mg injectate powder in 10 mL sterile water).
Give through a well-lubricated catheter.

Infusion: 50–150 µg/kg/min (0.2% solution).

Do not administer IV in a concentration greater than 1% (10 mg/mL).

Elimination: Hepatic.

How Supplied: Powder for injection: 500 mg, 2.5 g, 5.0 g with 50 mL, 250 mL, 500 mL diluent, respectively.

Dilution for Infusion: 500 mg in 250 mL D_5W or NS solution (2 mg/mL).

Pharmacology

A methylated oxybarbiturate that produces a rapid ultrashort-acting anesthesia. It depresses the sensory cortex, decreases motor activity, alters cerebellar function, and produces dose-dependent drowsiness, sedation, and hypnosis. These effects are thought to be mediated by enhanced γ-aminobutyric acid (GABA) actions in the CNS. GABA is thought to be a major inhibitory transmitter in the CNS. It does not produce analgesia and has no muscle relaxant properties. Methohexital may induce paradoxical excitement in elderly persons and children and in the presence of acute or chronic pain. It has a more rapid recovery of consciousness compared with thiopental. Induction may be accompanied by excitatory phenomenon (e.g., involuntary muscle movements). Cardiovascular effects are secondary to a decrease in myocardial contractility and peripheral vasodilation.

Pharmacokinetics

Onset of Action: IV, 20–40 sec. Rectal, <5 min.

Peak Effect: IV, 45 sec. Rectal, 5–10 min.

Duration of Action: IV, 5–10 min. Rectal, 30–90 min.

Interaction/Toxicity: Potentiates CNS and circulatory depressant effects of narcotics, sedative hypnotics, alcohol, volatile anesthetics; decreases effects of oral anticoagulants, digoxin, β-blockers, corticosteroids, quinidine, theophylline; actions prolonged by MAO inhibitors, chloramphenicol.

Guidelines/Precautions

1. Premedication with opioids reduces incidences of excitatory phenomenon.

2. Extravascular injection may cause necrosis, and intra-arterial injection may lead to gangrene. Treat the latter by injection in the artery (use subclavian artery if in spasm) of 10 mL 1% procaine or 40–80 mg dilute solution papaverine or local infiltration of phentolamine (2.5–5 mg in 10 mL) to produce vasodilation. Sympathectomy may be achieved by stellate ganglion or brachial plexus block.
3. Contraindicated in patients with latent or manifest porphyria.
4. Use with caution in patients in status asthmaticus.
5. Reduce dosage in elderly, hypovolemic, high-risk surgical patients and with concomitant use of narcotics and other sedative hypnotics.
6. Incompatible with lactated Ringer's solution and other acid solutions such as atropine sulfate, metocurine iodide, and succinylcholine chloride.

Principal Adverse Reactions

Cardiovascular: Myocardial depression, arrhythmias.
Pulmonary: Respiratory depression, laryngospasm, bronchospasm.
CNS: Emergence delirium, prolonged somnolence, headache.
GI: Nausea, emesis, hiccups.
Other: Rash, skeletal muscle hyperactivity, shivering.

METHOXAMINE HCL (VASOXYL)

Use(s): Vasoconstrictor; treatment of paroxysmal atrial tachycardia.
Dosing: IV: 1–5 mg. Give slowly. May repeat dose after 15 min.

IM: 5–15 mg (0.25 mg/kg) for prolonged effect.
Elimination: Hepatic.
How Supplied: Injection: 20 mg/mL.

Pharmacology

A selective α_1-receptor agonist that produces a prompt and prolonged rise in blood pressure by increasing peripheral resistance.

Already O-methylated and cannot be inactivated by COMT or metabolized by MAO and thus has a long duration of action. It has no direct effect on the heart and may produce reflex bradycardia secondary to increased systolic and diastolic blood pressures. Increased afterload decreases cardiac output in patients with heart failure.

Pharmacokinetics

Onset of Action: IV, almost immediate; IM, 15–20 min.
Peak Effect: IV, 0.5–2 min; IM, 15–20 min.
Duration of Action: IV, 15–60 min; IM, 60–90 min.
Interaction/Toxicity: Pressor effects potentiated with oxytocics, other sympathomimetic amines, and in patients receiving MAO inhibitors or tricyclic antidepressants; severe hypertensive response with concomitant administration of β-adrenergic-blocking agents, guanethidine, and reserpine; increases risk of cardiac arrhythmias during halothane anesthesia; extravasation may cause sloughing and necrosis.

Guidelines/Precautions

1. Use with extreme caution in elderly patients and patients with hyperthyroidism, bradycardia, partial heart block, myocardial disease, or severe arteriosclerosis.
2. Use is not a substitute for the replacement of blood, plasma, fluids, and electrolytes, which should be restored promptly when loss has occurred.
3. Infuse into large veins to prevent extravasation. Treat any extravasation with local infiltration of phentolamine (5–10 mg in 10 mL NS solution) or sympathetic block.
4. Contains sulfites and may cause allergic-type reactions (wheezing, anaphylaxis) in susceptible populations.

Principal Adverse Reactions

Cardiovascular: Reflex bradycardia, hypertension, hypotension.
Pulmonary: Respiratory distress.
CNS: Anxiety, tremors, dizziness, seizures, cerebral hemorrhage, headache.
GI: Projectile vomiting.
GU: Desire to void.

METHYLDOPA (ALDOMET, METHYLDOPATE)

Use(s): Antihypertensive.
Dosing: IV/PO, 250–500 mg bid or tid (20–40 mg/kg/day).
Elimination: Hepatic, renal.
How Supplied: Injection, 250 mg/5 mL; tablets, 125 mg, 250 mg, 500 mg; oral solution, 250 mg/5 mL.

Pharmacology

Methyldopa acts in the CNS to lower blood pressure. Once in the brain, the drug is converted to α-methylnorepinephrine by the enzyme dopa decarboxylase. α-methylnorepinephrine lowers arterial pressure through activation of α_2-adrenergic receptors and lowered sympathetic outflow.

Pharmacokinetics

Onset of Action: IV, 1–2 hr. PO, 3–6 hr.
Peak Effect: IV/PO, 4–6 hr.
Duration of Action: IV, 10–16 hr; PO, 12–24 hr.
Interaction/Toxicity: Reduces MAC for volatile anesthetics; false positive test result for pheochromocytoma; paradoxical hypertensive response with coadministration of propranolol (which blocks β_2-vasodilating component of α-methylnorepinephrine); dementia in patients who subsequently receive haloperidol; Coombs' positive test result for hemolytic anemia and liver dysfunction with prolonged therapy.

Guidelines/Precautions

1. Contraindicated in patients with active hepatic disease such as acute hepatitis or cirrhosis.
2. Paradoxical pressor response has been reported with IV methyldopa.

Principal Adverse Reactions

Cardiovascular: Bradycardia, paradoxical pressor response, hypotension, pericarditis.
CNS: Sedation, vertigo, headache, paresthesias, cerebrovascular insufficiency, Bell's palsy, choreoathetotic movements.
GI: Nausea, vomiting.
Hepatic: Jaundice, hepatitis, abnormal liver function test results.

Endocrine: Gynecomastia, lactation, amenorrhea.
Hematologic: Thrombocytopenia, hemolytic anemia; positive Coombs' test result.

METHYLENE BLUE (UROLENE BLUE)

Use(s): Treatment of drug-induced methemoglobinemia; dye effect to delineate body structures and fistulas and to confirm rupture of amniotic membranes; urinary antiseptic (oral route).
Dosing: IV, 1–2 mg/kg (inject over several minutes).
           PO, 65–130 mg tid after meals with a full glass of water. ·
Elimination: Renal.
How Supplied: Injection, 10 mg/mL; tablets, 55 mg, 65 mg.

Pharmacology

This compound has an oxidation-reduction action and a tissue-staining property. It has opposite actions on hemoglobin, depending on the concentration. In high concentrations, methylene blue converts the ferrous iron of reduced hemoglobin to the ferric form, and as a result, methemoglobin is produced. In contrast, low concentrations (recommended doses) are capable of hastening the conversion of methemoglobin to hemoglobin.

Pharmacokinetics

Onset of Action: IV, Almost immediate.
Peak Effect: IV, <1 hr.
Duration of Action: IV/PO, Varies.
Interaction/Toxicity: Discoloration of urine and feces; high concentrations in blood interfere with pulse oximetry, producing artifactual decrease in measured oxygen saturation (SaO_2); methemoglobin may alter measured oxygen saturation (falsely low at SaO_2 >85% and falsely high at SaO_2 <85%).

Guidelines/Precautions

1. Contraindicated in patients allergic to methylene blue, renal insufficiency, GGPD deficiency (hemolysis) and intraspinal injection. Do not use for methemoglobinemia in cyanide poisoning (releases free cyanide from cyanomethemoglobin).

2. Periodically monitor hemoglobin. Continued administration may cause marked anemia.
3. Slow IV injection to prevent local high concentration from producing additional methemoglobin.
4. Intra-amniotic injection may result in fetal tachycardia, neonatal hemolytic anemia, hyperbilirubinemia, methemoglobinemia, and blue skin.

Principal Adverse Reactions

Cardiovascular: Tachycardia, hypertension, precordial pain.
Pulmonary: Cyanosis.
CNS: Confusion, headache, dizziness.
GU: Bladder irritation.
GI: Nausea, vomiting, diarrhea, abdominal pain.
Dermatologic: Stains skin blue (may be removed by hypochlorite solution), necrotic abscesses.
Other: Methemoglobinemia, hemolytic anemia, hyperbilirubinemia.

METHYLERGONOVINE MALEATE (METHERGINE)

Use(s): Treatment of postpartum uterine atony and bleeding.
Dosing: IV/IM, 0.2 mg (give IV over 60 sec), repeat as required q2–4h; then PO, 0.2–0.4 mg q4–6h for 2–7 days.
Elimination: Hepatic.
How Supplied: Injection, 0.2 mg/mL; tablets, 0.2 mg.

Pharmacology

A semisynthetic ergot alkaloid that acts directly on the smooth muscle of the uterus and increases the tone, rate, and amplitude of rhythmic uterine contractions. Thus, it induces a rapid and sustained tetanic uterotonic effect that shortens the third stage of labor and reduces blood loss. The drug also constricts peripheral, mainly venous, capacitance vessels, raises CVP and blood pressure.

Pharmacokinetics

Onset: IV, immediate; IM, 2–5 min; PO, 5–15 min.
Peak Effect: IV <5 min; IM/PO, <30 min.
Duration: IV 45 min; IM/PO, >3 hr.

Interaction/Toxicity: Vasoconstriction potentiated by sympatho-mimetics such as ephedrine, phenylephrine, and nicotine.

Guidelines/Precautions

1. Use cautiously in patients with preeclampsia, hypertension, or cardiac disease.
2. Avoid in patients with peripheral vascular disease.
3. Discontinue if patients complain of tingling sensations in the extremities.
4. Inhibits lactation and is excreted in breast milk.

Principal Adverse Reactions

Cardiovascular: Hypertension, hypotension, chest pain.
Pulmonary: Dyspnea.
CNS: Dizziness, tinnitus, seizures, headache.
GI: Diarrhea, nausea, vomiting.
Other: Hematuria, thrombophlebitis, diaphoresis, gangrene of the fingers and toes.

METHYLPREDNISOLONE (MEDROL)
METHYLPREDNISOLONE SODIUM SUCCINATE (SOLU-MEDROL)*

Use(s): Anti-inflammatory, treatment of allergic reactions, short-term management of bronchodilator-unresponsive asthma and chronic obstructive pulmonary disease, steroid replacement, organ transplantation.

Dosing: (MEDROL):

    PO, 2–60 mg (0.117–1.66 mg/kg) daily in 4 divided doses. May be given as alternate doses to minimize side effects.

    (SOLU-MEDROL):

    IV/IM, 10 mg–1.5 g (0.03–30 mg/kg) daily.

        Usual dose, 10–250 mg. May be repeated up to 6 times daily.

        Life-threatening shock, IV, 30 mg/kg infused over 10–20 min every 4–6 hr if needed.

*For epidural precautions, see Bupivacaine, Guidelines/Precautions, item 10, p 20.

Intraarticular/intratissue, 4–80 mg. May repeat at
1–5 wk.

Epidural, 40–80 mg in 5–10 mL (preservative-free)
NS or local anesthetic. May repeat at 2–3 wk.

Elimination: Hepatic.[10]

How Supplied: Injection: 40 mg, 125 mg, 500 mg, 1000 mg,
2000 mg/vial; tablets: 2 mg, 4 mg, 8 mg, 16 mg, 24 mg, 32 mg.

Pharmacology

This methyl derivative of prednisolone is a potent anti-
inflammatory corticosteroid. Anti-inflammatory potency of 4 mg
of methylprednisolone is equivalent to that of 5 mg of prednisolone and 20 mg of cortisol. It has less tendency to cause salt and
water retention than prednisolone, hydrocortisone, or cortisone
and has a rapid onset but short duration of action. It may suppress
the hypothalamic-pituitary-adrenal axis.

Pharmacokinetics

Onset of Action: IV, Almost immediate.
Peak Effect: IV, <1 hr.
Duration of Action: IV, 12–36 hr.
Interaction/Toxicity: Clearance enhanced by phenytoin, phenobarbital, ephedrine, and rifampin; altered response to coumarin
anticoagulants; enhanced effect in patients with hypothyroidism
and cirrhosis; interacts with anticholinesterase agents (e.g., neostigmine) to produce severe weakness in patients with myasthenia
gravis; potassium-wasting effects enhanced with potassium-depleting diuretics (e.g., thiazides, furosemide); diminished response to toxoids and live or inactivated vaccines.

Guidelines/Precautions

1. Contraindicated in systemic fungal infections.
2. Use cautiously in patients with ocular herpes simplex for fear
   of corneal perforation.
3. After prolonged therapy, abrupt discontinuation may result in
   a withdrawal syndrome without evidence of adrenal insufficiency. To minimize morbidity associated with adrenal insufficiency, discontinue exogenous corticosteroid therapy gradually.
4. In patients on corticosteroid therapy subjected to any unusual
   stress, increased dosage of rapidly acting corticosteroid be-

fore, during, and after the stressful situation is indicated. Supplemental steroids should be empirically administered to all patients who have received daily steroid replacement for at least 1 wk in the year prior to surgery.
5. May mask signs of infection. There may be decreased resistance and inability of the host defense mechanisms to prevent dissemination of infection.

Principal Adverse Reactions

Cardiovascular: Arrhythmias, hypertension, congestive heart failure in susceptible patients.
CNS: Seizures, psychosis, increases intracranial pressure.
GI: Pancreatitis, peptic ulcer with perforation and hemorrhage.
Dermatologic: Impaired wound healing, petechiae, SLE-like syndrome.
Musculoskeletal: Weakness, myopathy, osteoporosis, aseptic necrosis.
Endocrine: Amenorrhea, growth suppression, hyperglycemia, negative nitrogen balance.
Fluid and Electrolyte Imbalances: Sodium and water retention, hypokalemia, metabolic alkalosis, hypocalcemia.
Intraspinal: Meningitis, arachnoiditis.
Other: Thromboembolism, diminishes response to toxoids and live or inactivated vaccines, increases susceptibility to and mask symptoms of infection.

METOCLOPRAMIDE (REGLAN)

Use(s): Stimulate gastric emptying, antiemetic, treatment of symptomatic gastroesophageal reflux and diabetic gastroparesis.
Dosing: IV/IM, 10 mg (give IV injection over 1–2 min).
PO, 10 mg 30 min before meals and at bedtime.
Elimination: Renal.
How Supplied: Injection, 5 mg/mL, 10 mg/mL; tablets, 5 mg, 10 mg; oral solution: 5 mg/5 mL.

Pharmacology

Metoclopramide is a derivative of procainamide. It stimulates motility of the upper GI tract and increases lower esophageal sphincter tone by 10–20 cm H_2O. Gastric acid secretion is not altered. Net effect is accelerated gastric emptying and intestinal transit. It sensitizes GI smooth muscle to the effects of acetylcholine and may cause release of acetylcholine from cholinergic nerve endings. Antiemetic effects may result from its antagonism of central and peripheral dopamine receptors and inhibition of chemoreceptor trigger zone–mediated vomiting. It produces minimal sedation and, rarely, may produce extrapyramidal reactions.

Pharmacokinetics

Onset of Action: IV, 1–3 min; IM, 10–15 min; PO, 30–60 min.
Peak Effect: IV/IM, <1 hr; PO, 1–2 hr.
Duration of Action: IV/IM/PO, 1–2 hr.
Interaction/Toxicity: Effects on GI motility antagonized by anticholinergic drugs and narcotic analgesics; sedative effects potentiated by alcohol, sedative hypnotics, tranquilizers, narcotics; diminishes absorption from the small bowel of tetracycline, acetaminophen, levodopa, ethanol; releases catecholamines in patients with essential hypertension and pheochromocytoma; intense feelings of anxiety and restlessness after rapid IV injection; extrapyramidal reactions.

Guidelines/Precautions

1. Use cautiously in patients with hypertension or those receiving MAO inhibitors. Metoclopramide-induced hypertensive crisis in patients with pheochromocytoma may be controlled with phentolamine.
2. Not recommended in children because of increased incidence of extrapyramidal reactions.
3. Contraindicated in patients with pheochromocytoma, epilepsy, GI hemorrhage, obstruction, or perforation or those receiving other drugs likely to cause extrapyramidal reactions.
4. Extrapyramidal reactions may consist of dystonic reactions, feelings of motor restlessness (akathisia), and parkinsonian signs and symptoms. Therapy should include discontinuation of metoclopramide or reduction in dosage and treatment with an anticholinergic antiparkinsonian agent (e.g., benztropine, trihexyphenidyl) or with diphenhydramine (IV/PO, 25 mg). Maintenance of an adequate airway should be instituted if necessary.

Principal Adverse Reactions

CVS: Hypertension, hypotension, arrhythmia.
CNS: Drowsiness, extrapyramidal reactions, akathisia, insomnia, anxiety.
GI: Nausea, diarrhea.
Other: Galactorrhea, gynecomastia, hypoglycemia.

METOCURINE IODIDE (METUBINE)

Use(s): Nondepolarizing muscle relaxant.
Dosing: Paralyzing, IV, 0.2–0.4 mg/kg.
Pretreatment/maintenance, IV, 0.04–0.07 mg/kg.
Elimination: Renal.
How Supplied: Injection: 2 mg/mL.

Pharmacology

A methyl analogue of tubocurarine that produces a nondepolarizing neuromuscular blockade at the myoneural junction. It does not produce autonomic ganglion blockade. Histamine release occurs less frequently than with *d*-tubocurarine and is related to dosage and rapidity of administration. Repeated doses may be accompanied by a cumulative effect. Effects on the cardiovascular system (e.g., changes in pulse rate, hypotension) are less than those reported with equipotent doses of tubocurarine and gallamine.

Pharmacokinetics

Onset of Action: <3 min.
Peak Effect: 3–5 min.
Duration of Action: 35–60 min.
Interaction/Toxicity: Effects potentiated by volatile anesthetics, aminoglycoside antibiotics, local anesthetics, quinidine, diuretics, magnesium, lithium, respiratory acidosis, hypokalemia; effects antagonized by anticholinesterase inhibitors such as neostigmine, edrophonium, pyridostigmine; resistance with concomitant use of phenytoin and in patients with burn injury and paresis; chemically incompatible with alkaline solutions, including solutions of barbiturate, meperidine, and morphine sulfate.

Guidelines/Precautions

1. Monitor response with peripheral nerve stimulator to minimize risk of overdosage.
2. Reverse effects with anticholinesterases such as pyridostigmine bromide, neostigmine, or edrophonium in conjunction with atropine or glycopyrrolate.
3. Rapid IV injection may produce hypotension, tachycardia, and signs of histamine release.
4. Pretreatment doses may induce a degree of neuromuscular blockade sufficient to cause hypoventilation in some patients.
5. Contraindicated in patients sensitive to iodide.

Principal Adverse Reactions

Cardiovascular: Hypotension.
Pulmonary: Hypoventilation, apnea, bronchospasm.
Musculoskeletal: Inadequate block, prolonged block.
Dermatologic: Erythema, flushing, anaphylactoid reactions.

METOPROLOL TARTRATE (LOPRESSOR)

Use(s): Antihypertensive, treatment of supraventricular, ventricular arrhythmias, and acute myocardial infarction; antianginal, symptomatic relief in thyrotoxic patients; adjunct treatment of alcohol withdrawal.
Dosing: Hypertension/angina: PO, 100–450 mg daily in single or divided doses (begin with 100 mg/day and increase at weekly intervals).

Acute myocardial infarction: early, IV, 15 mg (5 mg q2min for 3 doses), then PO, 50 mg q6h for 48 hr, then PO, 100 mg bid; patients intolerant of full IV dose, PO, 25–50 mg q6h; late treatment, PO, 100 mg bid.
Elimination: Hepatic.
How Supplied: Tablets, 50 mg, 100 mg; injection, 1 mg/mL.

Pharmacology

Metoprolol is a cardioselective β-blocker but can inhibit β_2-receptors in high doses. The mechanism for the antihypertensive effects of the drug is unknown. Reduced cardiac output, decreased renin release, or a central action may play a role. The antiarrhythmic effect is secondary to the reduction in sympathetic nervous system activity, whereas the antianginal effect reflects the decrease in myocardial oxygen consumption secondary to a reduction in heart rate and cardiac output.

Pharmacokinetics

Onset of Action: IV, almost immediate; PO, <15 min.
Peak Effect: IV, 20 min.
Duration of Action: IV/PO, 5–8 hr.
Interaction/Toxicity: Hypotensive effect potentiated by volatile anesthetics, catecholamine-depleting drugs (e.g., reserpine); may unmask negative inotropic effects of ketamine; prolongs elevation of plasma potassium after administration of succinylcholine; potentiates depolarizing and nondepolarizing muscle relaxants, e.g., succinylcholine, tubocurarine; may mask symptoms of hypoglycemia (e.g., tachycardia); increases serum levels of digoxin and morphine; rebound hypertension with abrupt withdrawal; may produce bradycardia, AV block, bronchospasm, and cardiac failure.

Guidelines/Precautions

1. Excessive myocardial depression may be treated with IV atropine (1–2 mg), IV isoproterenol (0.02–0.15 µg/kg/min), IV glucagon (1–5 mg), or a transvenous cardiac pacemaker.
2. Contraindicated in sinus bradycardia, heart block greater than first degree, cardiogenic shock, and overt failure.
3. Use with extreme caution, if at all, in patients with bronchospastic disease.
4. Increased risk of ischemia or infarction in patients with coronary artery disease if drug is withdrawn abruptly.

Principal Adverse Reactions

Cardiovascular: Hypotension, arrhythmias, rebound angina.
Pulmonary: Bronchospasm, dyspnea, cough.
CNS: Fatigue, depression, disorientation.
GI: Nausea, vomiting, pancreatitis.
Hematologic: Thrombocytopenic purpura.
Musculoskeletal: Arthralgia.

MIDAZOLAM HCL (VERSED)

Use(s): Premedication, amnesia, induction agent, supplementation of anesthesia.
Dosing: Sedation: IV, 0.5–5 mg (0.025–0.1 mg/kg). Titrate slowly to the desired effect, e.g., onset of slurred speech; continuously monitor respiratory and cardiac function); IM, 0.05–0.2 mg/kg; PO, 0.5–0.75 mg/kg (use high-potency injectate solution [5 mg/mL]; dilute in 3–5 mL apple juice or carbonated cola beverage; atropine, 0.03 mg/kg PO, may be added to reduce secretions); intranasal, 0.2–0.3 mg/kg (use high-potency injectate solution, [5 mg/mL]; rectal, 0.3–0.35 mg/kg (dilute in 5 mL NS solution).

Induction: IV, 50–350 μg/kg.
Infusion: 0.25–1.5 μg/kg/min.
Elimination: Renal.
How Supplied: Injection: 1 mg/mL, 5 mg/mL.
Dilution for Infusion: 15 mg in 250 mL D_5W or NS solution (60 μg/mL).

Pharmacology

This short-acting benzodiazepine possesses antianxiety, sedative, amnesic, anticonvulsant, and skeletal muscle relaxant properties. Neuromuscular transmission is not affected, and the action of nondepolarizing drugs is not altered. The mechanism of action is unknown, but it is thought to act by facilitating the effects of GABA like other benzodiazepine drugs. It depresses ventilation and decreases peripheral vascular resistance and blood pressure, especially in the presence of narcotic premedication, and/or hypovolemia. It has a more rapid onset, greater amnesic action, and a sedative potency 3–4 times that of diazepam. Slightly slower recovery compared with patients who received thiopental for induction. Predictable blood level–CNS response relationship.

Pharmacokinetics

Onset of Action: IV, 1–5 min; IM, 15 min; PO/rectal, <10 min; intranasal, <5 min.
Peak Effect: IV, 5–30 min; IM, 15–30 min; PO, 30 min; intranasal, 10 min; rectal, 20–30 min.

Duration of Action: IV/IM/PO/rectal, 2–6 hr.
Interaction/Toxicity: CNS and circulatory depressant effects potentiated by alcohol, narcotics, sedatives, volatile anesthetics; decreases MAC for volatile anesthetics, effects antagonized by flumazenil.

Guidelines/Precautions

1. Reduce doses in elderly, hypovolemic, high-risk patients and with concomitant use of other sedatives or narcotics.
2. Patients with chronic obstructive pulmonary disease (COPD) are unusually sensitive to the respiratory depressant effect.
3. Contraindicated in acute narrow-angle or open-angle glaucoma unless patients are receiving appropriate therapy.
4. Unexpected hypotension and respiratory depression may occur when given with opioids; consider smaller doses.
5. Respiratory depression and arrest may occur when used for conscious sedation. When used for conscious sedation, do not administer as a bolus. Treat overdose with supportive measures and flumazenil (slow IV, 0.2–1 mg).

Principal Adverse Reactions

Cardiovascular: Tachycardia, vasovagal episode, premature ventricular complexes, hypotension.
Pulmonary: Bronchospasm, laryngospasm, apnea, hypoventilation.
CNS: Euphoria, emergence delirium, prolonged emergence, tonic-clonic movements, agitation, hyperactivity.
GI: Salivation, retching, acid taste.
Dermatologic: Rash, pruritus, warmth or coldness at injection site.

MIVACURIUM CHLORIDE (MIVACRON)

Use(s): Nondepolarizing muscle relaxant.
Dosing: IV, paralyzing 0.07–0.2 mg/kg. (Children 0.1–0.2 mg/kg.) Administer over 5–15 sec.
  Pretreatment/maintenance, IV, 0.01–0.1 mg/kg.
  Infusion, 1–15 µg/kg/min.

Elimination: Plasma cholinesterase.
How Supplied: Injection: 2 mg/mL. Premixed Infusion: 0.5
mg/mL in 5% dextrose.
Dilution for Infusion: Inject solution: 25 mg in 50 mL D5W
or NS (0.5 mg/mL). Undiluted injectate solution (2 mg/mL) may
be used for infusion.

Pharmacology

This *bis*-benzylisoquinolinium diester compound is a short-acting
nondepolarizing neuromuscular blocking agent. It competes for
cholinergic receptors at the motor end plate. It is metabolized by
plasma cholinesterase and the duration of neuromuscular activity
is a third that of atracurium, half that of vecuronium, and 2 to 2.5
times that of succinylcholine. The time to onset of maximum effect is similar for recommended doses of mivacurium and intermediate-acting neuromuscular blockers, e.g., atracurium and vecuronium, but longer than that for succinylcholine. Unlike these
intermediate-acting agents, increasing the dosage of mivacurium
does not markedly increase the duration of action. Repeated doses
are not associated with tachyphylaxis and have minimal cumulative effect on duration of blockade. Higher doses (>0.2 mg/kg)
may be associated with decreases in mean arterial pressure, increases in heart rate, and elevation of plasma histamine concentrations.

Pharmacokinetics

Onset of Action: <2 min.
Peak Effect: 1–3 min.
Duration of Action: 6–10 min.
Interaction/Toxicity: Potentiated by prior administration of succinylcholine, volatile anesthetics, aminoglycoside, antibiotics, local anesthetics, loop diuretics, magnesium. lithium, ganglionic-
blocking drugs, hypothermia, hypokalemia, respiratory acidosis;
recurrent paralysis with quinidine; enhanced neuromuscular blockade in patients with low plasma cholinesterase, myasthenia gravis,
or inadequate adrenocortical function; increased sensitivity to mivacurium during pregnancy secondary to decreased pseudocholinesterase; effects antagonized by anticholinesterase inhibitors such
as neostigmine, edrophonium, pyridostigmine; increased resis-

tance or reversal of effects with use of theophylline and in patients with burn injury and paresis; incompatible with alkaline solutions having a pH greater than 8.5, e.g., barbiturate solutions.

Guidelines/Precautions

1. Monitor response with peripheral nerve stimulator to minimize risk of overdosage.
2. Reverse effects with anticholinesterases, such as pyridostigmine bromide, neostigmine, or edrophonium in conjunction with atropine or glycopyrrolate.
3. Pretreatment doses may induce a degree of neuromuscular blockade sufficient to cause hypoventilation in some patients.
4. Prolonged neuromuscular blockade may occur in patients with low plasma pseudocholinesterase, as in those with severe liver disease or cirrhosis, burns, malignant tumors, infections, decompensated heart disease, myxedema, peptic ulcer, pregnancy, dehydration, collagen disease, abnormal body temperatures, and patients receiving MAO inhibitors, oral contraceptives, glucocorticoids, or those with a recessive hereditary trait. Administer test doses of not more than 0.015–0.020 mg/kg of mivacurium.
5. Use with caution in patients with any history suggesting a greater sensitivity to the release of histamine or related mediators (e.g., asthma). Initial dose of mivacurium should be 0.15 mg/kg or less administered over 60 sec with adequate hydration and careful monitoring of hemodynamic status.
6. Initial dose requirements are higher in children and maintenance doses are generally required more frequently.
7. Contraindicated in patients known to have allergic hypersensitivity to mivacurium chloride or other benzylisoquinolinium agents. Use of mivacurium from multidose vials is contraindicated in patients with a known allergy to benzyl alcohol.

Principal Adverse Reactions

Cardiovascular: Hypotension, vasodilation, tachycardia, bradycardia.
Pulmonary: Hypoventilation, apnea, bronchospasm, laryngospasm, dyspnea.
Dermatologic: Rash, urticaria, erythema, injection site reaction.
Musculoskeletal: Inadequate block, prolonged block.

MORPHINE SULFATE (ASTRAMORPH, DURAMORPH, MORPHINE, MS CONTIN)*

Use(s): Premedication, analgesia, anesthesia, treatment of pain associated with myocardial ischemia and dyspnea associated with acute left ventricular failure and pulmonary edema.

Dosing: Analgesia: IV, 2.5–15 mg (children, 0.05–0.2 mg/kg, maximum dose, 15 mg); IM/SC, 2.5–20 mg (children, 0.05–0.2 mg/kg, maximum dose, 15 mg); PO, 10–30 mg q4h prn for pain; PO, extended release, 30 mg q12h; rectal, 10–20 mg q4h; intraarticular, 0.5–1 mg (dilute in 40 mL NS or 0.025% bupivacaine); induction IV, 1 mg/kg; epidural (bolus), 2–5 mg (40–100 μg/kg), epidural (infusion), 0.1–1 mg/hr (2–20 μg/kg/hr). Use preservative-free solution); spinal, 0.2–1 mg (4–20 μg/kg/hr). Use preservative-free solution).

Patient-controlled analgesia: IV (bolus), 0.5–3.0 mg; (infusion), 0.5–2.0 mg/hr; (lockout interval), 5–20 min; epidural (bolus), 0.1 mg; (infusion), 0.4 mg/hr; lockout interval, 10 min.

Elimination: Hepatic.

How Supplied: Injection: 0.5 mg/mL, 1 mg/mL, 2 mg/mL, 3 mg/mL, 4 mg/mL, 5 mg/mL, 8 mg/mL, 10 mg/mL, 15 mg/mL; preservative-free injection: 0.5 mg/mL, 1 mg/mL; tablets: 10 mg, 15 mg, 30 mg; tablets (extended release): 30 mg, 60 mg; oral solution: 10 mg/5 mL, 20 mg/mL, 20 mg/5 mL, 100 mg/5 mL; rectal suppositories: 5 mg, 10 mg, 20 mg, 30 mg.

Dilution for Infusion: IV, 20 mg in 100 mL NS (0.2 mg/mL); epidural, 10 mg in 100 mL local anesthetic or (preservative-free) NS solution (0.1 mg/mL).

Pharmacology

This alkaloid of opium exerts its primary effects on the CNS and organs containing smooth muscle. It produces analgesia, drowsiness, euphoria, dose-related depression of respiration, interference with adrenocortical response to stress (at high doses), and reduction in peripheral resistance (arteriolar and venous dilation), with little or no effect on cardiac index. Constipating effects of mor-

*For epidural/intrathecal precautions, see Alfentanil, Guidelines/Precautions, items 5 and 6, pp 4–5.

phine result from induction of nonpropulsive contractions through the GI tract. Depression of the cough reflex is by a direct effect on the cough centers in the medulla. It releases histamine, which can cause pruritus and/or bronchospasm. It may induce nausea and vomiting by activating the chemoreceptor trigger zone.

Pharmacokinetics

Onset of Action: IV, almost immediate; IM, 1–5 min; PO, <60 min; epidural and spinal, 15–60 min.
Peak Effect: IV, 5–20 min; IM, 30–60 min; SC, 50–90 min; PO, <60 min; rectal, 20–60 min; epidural/spinal, 30 min.
Duration of Action: IV/IM/SC, 2–7 hr; epidural/spinal, 6–24 hr.
Interaction/Toxicity: CNS and cardiovascular depressant effects potentiated by alcohol, sedatives, antihistamines, phenothiazines, butyrophenones, MAO inhibitors, and tricyclic antidepressants; may decrease the effect of diuretics in patients with CHF; analgesia enhanced by α_2-agonists, e.g., clonidine.

Guidelines/Precautions

1. Reduce dose in elderly, hypovolemic, or high-risk surgical patients and with concomitant use of sedatives and other narcotics.
2. The narcotic antagonist naloxone is a specific antidote (IV, ≥0.2–0.4 mg). Reversal of narcotic effect may lead to onset of pain and release of catecholamines.
3. Crosses the placental barrier; usage in labor may produce depression of respiration in the neonate. Resuscitation may be required; have naloxone available.
4. Incidences of reactivation of herpes simplex have occurred after epidural or spinal administration of morphine.

Principal Adverse Reactions

Cardiovascular: Hypotension, hypertension, bradycardia, arrhythmias, chest wall rigidity.
Pulmonary: Bronchospasm, laryngospasm.
CNS: Blurred vision, syncope, euphoria, dysphoria.
GU: Urinary retention, antidiuretic effect, ureteral spasm.
GI: Biliary tract spasm, constipation, anorexia, nausea, vomiting.
Allergic: Pruritus, urticaria.
Musculoskeletal: Chest wall rigidity.

NALBUPHINE HCL (NUBAIN)

Use(s): Analgesia; anesthesia.
Dosing: Sedation and analgesia: IV/IM/SC, 5–10 mg (0.1–0.3
        mg/kg).
        Induction: IV, 0.3–3 mg/kg.
        Patient-controlled analgesia: IV (bolus), 1–5 mg; lock-
        out interval, 5–15 min.
Elimination: Hepatic.
How Supplied: Injection: 10 mg/mL, 20 mg/mL.

Pharmacology

A synthetic opioid agonist-antagonist (partial agonist) and a potent
analgesic. It is related chemically to oxymorphone and naloxone.
Nalbuphine is equal in potency as an analgesic to morphine and
one fourth as potent as nalorphine as an antagonist. It exhibits
ceiling effect at high doses (>30 mg) for respiratory depression
and analgesia. Cardiovascular stability is good.

Pharmacokinetics

Onset of Action: IV, 2–3 min; IM/SC, <15 min.
Peak Effect: IV, 5–15 min.
Duration of Action: IV/IM/SC, 3–6 hr.
Interaction/Toxicity: In nondependent patients, potentiates depressant effect of other narcotics, volatile anesthetics, sedative
hypnotics, phenothiazines; precipitates withdrawal symptoms in
narcotic-dependent patients; may produce pruritus, bronchospasm,
hypotension, hypertension.

Guidelines/Precautions

1. Reduce dose in elderly, hypovolemic, or high-risk surgical
   patients and with concomitant use of sedatives and other narcotics.
2. Naloxone is a specific antidote (IV, ≥0.2–0.4 mg).
3. May worsen gallbladder pain.
4. Crosses the placental barrier; usage in labor may produce depression of respiration in the neonate. Resuscitation may be
   required; have naloxone available.
5. Use with caution in patients who have been chronically re-

ceiving opiate agonists. High doses may precipitate with-drawal symptoms as a result of opiate antagonist effect.

Principal Adverse Reactions

Cardiovascular: Hypertension, hypotension, bradycardia, tachy-cardia.
Pulmonary: Respiratory depression, dyspnea, asthma.
CNS: Euphoria, dysphoria, confusion, sedation.
GI: Cramps, dyspepsia, bitter taste.
Dermatologic: Itching, burning, urticaria.
Other: Speech difficulty, urinary urgency, blurred vision, flush-ing.

NALOXONE HCL (NARCAN)

Use(s): Reversal of narcotic depression.
Dosing: IV/IM/SC, 0.1–2 mg (10–40 μg/kg), titrate to patient response; may repeat at 2- to 3-min intervals; re-sponse should occur with a maximum dose of 10 mg.
Elimination: Hepatic.
How Supplied: Injection, 0.4 mg/mL, 1 mg/mL; neonatal injec-tion: 0.02 mg/mL.

Pharmacology

This drug is a pure opioid antagonist with no agonist activity. It competitively inhibits opiate agonists at μ-, δ-, and κ-receptor sites and prevents or reverses the effects of opioids, including res-piratory depression, sedation, and hypotension. Naloxone can also reverse the psychotomimetic and dysphoric effects of agonists-antagonists such as pentazocine. It does not produce respiratory depression, psychotomimetic effects, or pupillary constriction. It shows no pharmacologic activity in the absence of narcotics and produces withdrawal symptoms in the presence of physical depen-dence.

Pharmacokinetics

Onset of Action: IV, 1–2 min; IM/SC, 2–5 min.
Peak Effect: IV/IM/SC, 5–15 min.

Duration of Action: IV/IM/SC, 1–4 hr.
Interaction/Toxicity: Reversal of analgesia; increased sympathetic nervous system activity, including tachycardia, hypertension, pulmonary edema, and cardiac arrhythmias; nausea and vomiting related to dose and speed of injection.

Guidelines/Precautions

1. Use with caution in patients with preexisting cardiac disease or who have received potentially cardiotoxic drugs.
2. Titrate slowly to desired effect. Excessive dosage of naloxone may result in reversal of analgesia and other significant side effects (hypertension, excitement, acute pulmonary edema, cardiac arrhythmias).
3. Patients who have responded to naloxone should be carefully monitored because the duration of action of some opiates may exceed that of naloxone. Repeated doses of naloxone should be administered to those patients when necessary.
4. Administer cautiously to persons who are known or suspected to be physically dependent on opioids, including newborns of mothers with narcotic dependence. Reversal of narcotic effects will precipitate acute abstinence syndrome.

Principal Adverse Reactions

Cardiovascular: Tachycardia, hypertension, hypotension, arrhythmias.
Pulmonary: Pulmonary edema.
CNS: Tremulousness, reversal of analgesia, seizures.
GI: Nausea, vomiting.
Other: Sweating.

NEOSTIGMINE (PROSTIGMIN)

Use(s): Reversal of nondepolarizing muscle relaxants; treatment of myasthenia gravis, postoperative ileus, urinary retention.
Dosing: Reversal: slow IV, 0.05 mg/kg (maximum dose, 5 mg), with atropine, 0.015 mg/kg, or glycopyrrolate, 0.01 mg/kg.
Myasthenia gravis: PO, 15–375 mg daily (3 divided doses); or IM/slow IV, 0.5–2 mg (dose must be individualized).

Postoperative ileus/urinary retention: IM/SC, 0.25–1
mg q4–6h.

Elimination: Hepatic, plasma esterases.

How Supplied: Injection: 0.25 mg/mL (1:4000), 0.5 mg/mL
(1:2000), 1 mg/mL (1:1000); tablets: 15 mg.

Pharmacology

Neostigmine inhibits the hydrolysis of acetylcholine by competing
with acetylcholine for attachment to acetylcholinesterase at the es-
teratic site. Buildup of acetylcholine facilitates the transmission of
impulses across the neuromuscular junction. In myasthenia gravis
there is an increased response of skeletal muscle to repetitive impulses because of increased availability of acetylcholine. Cholinergic stimulation is useful in treating postoperative ileus. When
used for reversal of neuromuscular blockade, the muscarinic cholinergic effects (bradycardia, salivation) may be prevented by concurrent use of atropine or glycopyrrolate.

Pharmacokinetics

Onset of Action: Reversal: IV, <3 min. Myaesthenia IM, <20
min. Myasthenia PO, 45–75 min.

Peak Effect: Reversal: 3–14 min (twitch height >20% control).
Reversal: 8–29 min (twitch height <20% control). Myaesthenia
IM, 20–30 min.

Duration of Action: Reversal: IV, 40–60 min. Myaesthenia IM/
PO, 2–4 hr.

Interaction/Toxicity: Does not antagonize and may prolong the
phase 1 block of depolarizing muscle relaxants such as succinylcholine; antagonizes the effects of nondepolarizing muscle relaxants such as tubocurarine, atracurium, vecuronium, and pancuronium; antagonism of neuromuscular blockade is reduced by
aminoglycoside antibiotics, hypothermia, hypokalemia, respiratory, and metabolic acidosis.

Guidelines/Precautions

1. Contraindicated in patients with peritonitis or mechanical obstruction of the intestines or urinary tract.
2. Neostigmine overdosage may induce a cholinergic crisis characterized by nausea, vomiting, bradycardia or tachycardia,
   excessive salivation and sweating, bronchospasm, weakness,
   and paralysis.

3. Treatment of a cholinergic crisis includes discontinuation of neostigmine and administration of atropine (10 μg/kg IV q3–10min until muscarinic symptoms disappear), and, if necessary, pralidoxime (15 mg/kg IV over 2 min) for reversal of nicotinic symptoms. Give other supportive treatment as indicated (artificial respiration, tracheostomy, oxygen etc).
4. Use with caution in patients with bradycardia, bronchial asthma, epilepsy, cardiac arrhythmias, or peptic ulcer.

Principal Adverse Reactions

Cardiovascular: Bradycardia, tachycardia, AV block, nodal rhythm, hypotension.
Pulmonary: Increased oral, pharyngeal and bronchial secretions, bronchospasm, respiratory depression.
CNS: Seizures, dysarthria, headaches.
GI: Nausea, emesis, flatulence, increased peristalsis.
GU: Urinary frequency.
Dermatologic: Rash, urticaria.
Allergic: Allergic reactions, anaphylaxis.

NIFEDIPINE (ADALAT, PROCARDIA)

Use(s):   Antiangina/antihypertensive, suppressor of preterm labor.
Dosing: Angina/hypertension: PO, 10–20 mg tid (maximum dose, 180 mg/day). PO (sustained release) (PO-SR), 30–60 mg once daily.

Unlabeled route: Sublingual (puncture capsule, apply contents sublingually) or intrabuccal (puncture capsule 10 times, chew).

Preterm labor: Sublingual, 10 mg q 20 min until cessation of contractions (max. dose, 40 mg in 1 hr) then PO, 20 mg q8h for 3 days.
Elimination: Hepatic, renal.
How Supplied: Capsules: 10 mg, 20 mg; tablets (SR): 30 mg, 60 mg, 90 mg.

Pharmacology

Nifedipine is a dihydropyridine calcium channel blocker. It inhibits the transmembrane influx of calcium ions into cardiac muscle and smooth muscle. It possesses greater coronary and peripheral arterial vasodilator properties than verapamil and minimal effects on venous capacitance. It has little or no direct depressant effect on SA or AV node activity and, consequently, may be used safely in patients with low heart rate. The antihypertensive effects are probably caused by decreased peripheral vascular resistance. A reflex increase in heart rate, cardiac output, and fluid retention from peripheral vasodilation may offset the antihypertensive effect. Nifedipine improves myocardial oxygen supply and demand balance, which accounts for its effectiveness in the treatment of angina pectoris.

Pharmacokinetics

Onset of Action: PO, 20 min; sublingual, 5 min.
Peak Effect: PO, 30 min; PO-SR, 6 hr; sublingual, 20–45 min.
Duration of Action: PO/sublingual, 4–12 hr; PO-SR, 24 hr.
Interaction/Toxicity: Potentiates effects of depolarizing and nondepolarizing muscle relaxants; additive cardiovascular depressant effects with use of volatile anesthetics, other antihypertensives such as diuretics, ACE inhibitors, vasodilators; increases toxicity of digoxin, benzodiazepines, carbamazepine, oral hypoglycemics, and possibly quinidine and theophylline; cardiac failure, AV conduction disturbances, and sinus bradycardia with concurrent use of β-blockers; severe hypotension and bradycardia may occur with bupivacaine; concomitant use of IV verapamil and IV dantrolene may result in cardiovascular collapse; decreases lithium effect and neurotoxicity; decreased clearance with cimetidine; chemically incompatible with solutions of bicarbonate or nafcillin; may be displaced or displace from binding sites other highly protein-bound drugs such as oral anticoagulants, hydantoins, salicylates, sulfonamides, and sulfonylureas.

Guidelines/Precautions

1. Careful monitoring of blood pressure during initial administration and titration of nifedipine.
2. Use with caution in the elderly, hypovolemic patients, and those with acute MI or unstable angina.
3. Do not chew or divide SR tablets.

Principal Adverse Reactions

Cardiovascular: Hypotension, palpitations, peripheral edema.
Pulmonary: Bronchospasm, shortness of breath, nasal and chest congestion.
CNS: Headache, dizziness, nervousness.

GI: Nausea, diarrhea, constipation.
Musculoskeletal: Inflammation, joint stiffness, peripheral edema.
Dermatologic: Pruritus, urticaria.
Other: Fever, chills, sweating.

NITROGLYCERIN (NITROL, NITROSTAT, TRIDIL, NITROCINE, NITROLIN, NITROGLYN, NITRO-BID, TRANSDERM-NITRO, NITRODISC, AND OINTMENT)

Use(s): Controlled hypotension, antianginal, treatment of pulmonary edema and CHF associated with acute myocardial infarction.
Dosing: IV infusion: 5–200 μg/min (0.1–4 μg/kg/min) (absorbed in plastic and polyvinyl chloride [PVC] tubings; use glass bottle and supplied infusion set).

Tablets (Sublingual): 0.15–0.6 mg q5min prn to maximum of 3 doses in 15 min; (SR-buccal): 1–2 mg q3–5h (place tablet between lip and gum above incisors); (PO-SR): 1.3–9 mg q8–12h prn.

Capsules (PO-SR): 1.3–9 mg q8–12h prn.

Ointment: ½–2 in. q8h (maximum dose, 4–5 in. q4h).

Transdermal systems: Apply pad once daily. Titrate to a higher dose strength as needed for optimal effect.

Aerosol: 1–2 metered dose on oral mucosa. Maximum, 3 doses in 15min.

Elimination: Hepatic, renal.
How Supplied: Injection: 0.5 mg/mL, 0.8 mg/mL, 5 mg/mL, 10 mg/mL. Tablets: Sublingual, 0.15 mg (1/400 gr), 0.3 mg (1/200 gr), 0.4 mg (1/150 gr), 0.6 mg (1/100 gr); SR-buccal, 1 mg, 2 mg, 3 mg; PO-SR, 2.5 mg, 2.6 mg, 6.5 mg, 9 mg. Capsules: PO-SR, 2.5 mg, 6.5 mg, 9 mg. Aerosol: translingual, 0.4 mg/metered dose. Transdermal systems: 2.5 mg/24hr, 5 mg/24hr, 7.5 mg/24hr, 10 mg/24hr, 15 mg/24hr. Ointment: 2% (1 in. contains 15 mg nitroglycerin).
Dilution for Infusion: 8-mg vial: Dilute in 250 mL D_5W or NS solution (32 μg/mL). 50 mg vial: Dilute in 250 ml D_5W or NS solution (200 μg/mL). 100 mg vial: Dilute in 250 mL D_5W or NS solution (400 μg/mL).

Pharmacology

This organic nitrate produces a vasodilator effect principally on venous capacitance vessels. This produces peripheral pooling of blood, decreasing venous return, reducing left ventricular end-diastolic pressure (preload) and ventricular size. The decreased diameter of the left ventricle reduces wall tension according to the law of Laplace and decreases cardiac work. At higher doses, arteriolar relaxation reduces systemic vascular resistance and arterial pressure (afterload). All of these factors help improve myocardial oxygen supply/demand ratio. The drug also causes the redistribution of blood to ischemic areas of the subendocardium in angina pectoris and may decrease area of damage in myocardial infarction. Nitroglycerin may alter pulmonary ventilation/perfusion ratio and increase cerebral blood flow.

Pharmacokinetics

Onset of Action: IV, 1–2 min; sublingual, 1–3 min; PO-SR, 20–45 min; transdermal, 40–60 min.
Peak Effect: IV, 1–5 min.
Duration of Action: IV, 3–5 min; sublingual, 30–60 min; PO-SR, 3–8 hr; transdermal, 18–24 hr; aerosol translingual, 30–60 min.
Interaction/Toxicity: Hypotensive effects potentiated by alcohol, phenothiazines, calcium channel blockers, β-adrenergic blockers, other nitrates, nitrites, and antihypertensives; may antagonize the anticoagulant effect of heparin; methemoglobinemia at high doses.

Guidelines/Precautions

1. Use cautiously in patients with hypotension, uncorrected hypovolemia, increased intracranial pressure, constrictive pericarditis and pericardial tamponade, and inadequate cerebral circulation.
2. Infusion pumps may fail to occlude the non-PVC infusion sets completely because the non-PVC tubing is less pliable than standard PVC tubing used. The results may be excessive flow at low infusion rate settings, causing alarms or unregulated gravity flow when the infusion pump is stopped. This could lead to overinfusion.
3. Methemoglobinemia may be caused by high doses of nitrites,

especially in individuals with methemoglobin reductase deficiency. Treat with high-flow oxygen and administer methylene blue slowly IV at a dose of 0.1–0.2 mL/kg (1–2 mg/kg).

4. Nitroglycerin transdermal systems should be removed from the site(s) of application before defibrillation or cardioversion is attempted because altered electrical conductivity and enhanced potential for arching may occur.

5. Due to alcohol present in IV nitroglycerin solutions, prolonged administration of high doses may result in mild alcoholic intoxication.

Principal Adverse Reactions

Cardiovascular: Tachycardia, palpitations, hypotension, paradoxical bradycardia and increased angina, collapse.
CNS: Headache, dizziness, vertigo.
GI: Nausea, vomiting, abdominal pain.
Dermatologic: Flushing, exfoliative or contact dermatitis.
Other: Methemoglobinemia.

NOREPINEPHRINE BITARTRATE (LEVOPHED)

Use(s): Vasoconstrictor, inotrope.
Dosing: Infusion, 2–20 μg/min (0.04–0.4 μg/kg/min).
Elimination: Enzymatic degradation.
How Supplied: Injection, 1 mg/mL.
Dilution for Infusion: 8 mg in 500 mL D_5W (16 μg/mL).

Pharmacology

This catecholamine produces potent peripheral vasoconstrictor actions on both arterial and venous vascular beds (α-adrenergic action). It is a potent inotropic stimulator of the heart (β_1-adrenergic action) but to a lesser degree than epinephrine or isoproterenol. Norepinephrine does not stimulate β_2-adrenergic receptors of the bronchi or peripheral blood vessels. Systolic and diastolic blood pressures and coronary artery blood flow are increased. Cardiac output varies reflexly with systemic hypertension but is usually increased in hypotensive subjects when blood pressure is raised to an optimal level. On other occasions, increased baroreceptor activity reflexly decreases the heart rate. The drug reduces renal, hepatic, cerebral, and muscle blood flow.

Pharmacokinetics

Onset of Action: < 1 min.
Peak Effect: 1–2 min.
Duration of Action: 2–10 min.
Interaction/Toxicity: Increased risk of arrhythmias with use of volatile anesthetics or bretylium or in patients with profound hypoxia or hypercarbia; pressor effect potentiated in patients receiving MAO inhibitors, tricyclic antidepressants, guanethidine, oxytocics; necrosis or gangrene with extravasation.

Guidelines/Precautions

1. Administer into large vein to minimize extravasation. Treat extravasation immediately with local infiltration of phentolamine (5–10 mg in 10 mL NS solution) or sympathetic block.
2. Use is not a substitute for the replacement of blood, plasma, fluids, and electrolytes, which should be restored promptly when loss has occurred.
3. Contraindicated in patients with mesenteric or peripheral vascular thrombosis.

Principal Adverse Reactions

Cardiovascular: Bradycardia, tachyarrhythmias, hypertension, decreased cardiac output.
CNS: Headache.
Other: Plasma volume depletion.

ONDANSETRON HCl (ZOFRAN INJECTION)

Use(s): Prevention of postoperative nausea and/or vomiting. For patients who have nausea and/or vomiting postoperatively, ZOFRAN® (ondansetron HCl) Injection may be given to prevent further episodes. As with other antiemetics, routine prophylaxis is not recommended for patients in whom there is little expectation that nausea and/or vomiting will occur postoperatively. When nausea and/or vomiting must be avoided in patients postoperatively, ZOFRAN® (ondansetron HCl) Injection is recommended even when the incidence of postoperative nausea and/or vomiting is low. For patients who have nausea and/or vomiting postoperatively, ZOFRAN Injection may be given to prevent further episodes.

Prevention of nausea and vomiting associated with initial and repeat courses of emetogenic cancer chemotherapy, including high-dose cisplatin. (For further information, please consult complete Prescribing Information for ZOFRAN Injection on last pages of this book.)

Dosing: Prevention of postoperative nausea and/or vomiting: **NO DILUTION NECESSARY.** Immediately before induction of anesthesia, or postoperatively if the patient experiences nausea and/or vomiting occurring shortly after surgery, administer 4 mg **undiluted** intravenously in not less than 30 seconds, preferably over 2 to 5 minutes. Repeat dosing for patients who continue to experience nausea and/or vomiting postoperatively has not been studied. While recommended as a fixed dose for all, few patients weighing more than 80 kg or less than 40 kg have been studied.

Elimination: Hepatic.

How Supplied: Injection: 2 mg/mL is supplied in 2-mL single-dose vials and 20-mL multidose vials.

Pharmacology

Ondansetron is a selective 5-HT$_3$ receptor antagonist. 5-HT$_3$ receptors are present both peripherally on vagal nerve terminals and centrally in the chemoreceptor trigger zone of the area postrema. Ondansetron may antagonize the emetic effects of serotonin at either or both receptor sites. Ondansetron does not antagonize dopamine receptors.

Pharmacokinetics

Duration of Action: The mean half-life of 3.6 hours in normal patients increased to 9.2 hours in patients with mild to moderate hepatic impairment and was prolonged to 20.6 hours in patients with severe hepatic insufficiency.

Interaction: Ondansetron does not itself appear to induce or inhibit the cytochrome P-450 drug-metabolizing enzyme system of the liver. Because ondansetron is metabolized by hepatic cytochrome P-450 drug-metabolizing enzymes, inducers or inhibitors of these enzymes may change the clearance and, hence, the half-life of ondansetron. On the basis of limited available data, no dosage adjustment is recommended for patients on these drugs.

Guidelines/Precautions:

1. Ondansetron does not stimulate gastric or intestinal peristalsis. It should not be used in place of a nasogastric tube. As with other antiemetics, the use of ondansetron in abdominal surgery may mask a progressive ileus and/or gastric distention.
2. It is not known whether ondansetron is excreted in human milk. Caution should be exercised when ondansetron is administered to a nursing woman.
3. Dosage adjustment is not needed in patients over the age of 65. In clinical trials with patients with cancer, there was neither a difference in safety nor efficacy in patients over 65 years of age or under 65 years of age.
4. There is no experience with the use of ZOFRAN Injection in the prevention or treatment of postoperative nausea and vomiting in children.

Principal Adverse Reactions

CNS: Headache, dizziness, drowsiness/sedation.

Musculoskeletal: Pain, shivers.

In clinical trials, rates of these events were not significantly different in the ondansetron and placebo groups.

OXYTOCIN (PITOCIN, SYNTOCINON)

Use(s): Improvement of uterine contractions, control of postpartum hemorrhage.
Dosing: Antepartum: Infusion, 1–20 mU/min.
  Postpartum: Infusion, 20–40 mU/min (titrate to control uterine atony); IV bolus, 0.6–1.8 units; IM, 3–10 units.
Elimination: Hepatic.
How Supplied: Injection, 10 units/mL; nasal solution, 40 units/mL.
Dilution for Infusion: 10–40 units in 1 L NS solution (10–40 mU/mL).

Dilution for Infusion: 10–40 units in 1 L NS solution (10–40 mU/mL).

Pharmacology

This naturally occurring nonapeptide hormone stimulates uterine smooth muscle contractions. It increases both the force and frequency of existing rhythmic contractions and raises the tone of the uterine musculature. The sensitivity of the uterus to oxytocin increases gradually during gestation and sharply immediately before parturition. The hormone is structurally similar to ADH and may produce water intoxication. High doses produce a marked but transient vasodilation, hypotension, and flushing, accompanied by a reflex tachycardia and increased cardiac output.

Pharmacokinetics

Onset of Action: IV, almost immediate; IM, 3–5 min.
Peak Effect: IV, <20 min; IM, 40 min.
Duration of Action: IV, 20 min–1 hr; IM, 2–3 hr.
Interaction/Toxicity: Potentiates pressor effects of sympathomimetics (e.g., ephedrine, phenylephrine).

Guidelines/Precautions

1. When oxytocin is used for induction or stimulation of labor, administer only by the IV route.
2. Monitor uterine activity and fetal heart rate throughout the infusion of oxytocin. Discontinue infusion in event of uterine hyperactivity or fetal distress and administer oxygen to the mother, who should be put in the lateral position.
3. When oxytocin is administered by continuous infusion, monitor fluid intake to minimize risk of water intoxication.
4. Contraindicated in significant cephalopelvic disproportion, in fetal distress where delivery is not imminent, and when vaginal delivery is contraindicated.
5. Use cautiously in patients with preeclampsia, essential hypertension, or cardiac disease.

Principal Adverse Reactions

Cardiovascular: Arrhythmia, hypotension, hypertension, tachycardia.
CNS: Subarachnoid hemorrhage.

GI: Nausea, vomiting.
Allergic: Anaphylactic reactions, flushing.
Uterus: Hypertonicity, spasm, rupture.
Fetal: Bradycardia, arrhythmias, brain damage, low Apgar scores at 5 min.
Other: Afibrinogenemia, water retention, hyponatremia.

PANCURONIUM BROMIDE (PAVULON)

Use(s): Nondepolarizing muscle relaxant.
Dosing: IV (paralyzing), 0.04–0.1 mg/kg.
  Pretreatment/maintenance, 0.01–0.02 mg/kg.
Elimination: Renal, hepatic.
How Supplied: Injection: 1 mg/mL, 2 mg/mL.

Pharmacology

This synthetic bisquaternary amino corticosteroid is a long-acting nondepolarizing neuromuscular blocking agent. It acts by competing for cholinergic receptors at the motor end plate. The increased heart rate may result from vagolytic actions on the heart. Increased mean arterial pressure and cardiac output may occur by an activation of the sympathetic nervous system and inhibition of catecholamine reuptake. Histamine release rarely occurs.

Pharmacokinetics

Onset of Action: 1–3 min.
Peak Effect: 3–5 min.
Duration of Action: 40–65 min.
Interaction/Toxicity: Potentiated by prior administration of succinylcholine, volatile anesthetics, aminoglycoside antibiotics, local anesthetics, loop diuretics, magnesium, lithium, ganglionic blocking drugs, hypothermia, hypokalemia, respiratory acidosis; increases risk of arrhythmia in patients receiving tricyclic antidepressants and volatile anesthetics; recurrent paralysis with quinidine, enhanced neuromuscular blockade in patients with myasthenia gravis or inadequate adrenocortical function; effects antagonized by anticholinesterase inhibitors such as neostigmine, edrophonium, pyridostigmine; increased resistance or reversal of

effects with use of theophylline and in patients with burn injury and paresis.

Guidelines/Precautions

1. Monitor response with peripheral nerve stimulator to minimize risk of overdosage.
2. Reverse effects with anticholinesterases such as pyridostigmine bromide, neostigmine, or edrophonium in conjunction with atropine or glycopyrrolate.
3. Pretreatment doses may induce a degree of neuromuscular blockade sufficient to cause hypoventilation in some patients.

Principal Adverse Reactions

Cardiovascular: Tachycardia, hypertension.
Pulmonary: Hypoventilation, apnea, bronchospasm.
GI: Salivation.
Allergic: Flushing, anaphylactoid reactions.
Musculoskeletal: Inadequate block, prolonged block.

PHENTOLAMINE (REGITINE)

Use(s): Arterial dilator, controlled hypotension, treatment of acute hypertensive crises that may accompany intraoperative manipulation of a pheochromocytoma or autonomic hyperreflexia, prevention or treatment of dermal necrosis and sloughing after IV administration or extravasation of a barbiturate or sympathomimetic.

Dosing: Antihypertensive: IV/IM, 2.5–5 mg (0.05–0.1 mg/kg);
Infusion: 0.1–1 mg/min (10–20 µg/kg/min).
Antisloughing infiltration: 5–10 mg (0.1–0.2 mg/kg).
Maximum dose, 10 mg. Dilute in 10 mL NS solution.
Elimination: Hepatic.
How Supplied: Injection: 5 mg/mL.
Dilution for Infusion: 200 mg in 100 mL D_5W or NS solution (2 mg/mL).

Pharmacology

Phentolamine is an imidazoline sympathomimetic that blocks both α_1- and α_2-adrenergic receptors in the periphery. It produces peripheral vasodilation. Blockade of autoregulatory, pre-synaptic α_2-receptors leads to enhanced neuronal release of norepinephrine from catecholaminergic neurons. This action may enhance the positive inotropic and chronotropic effects produced by phentolamine stimulation of β-adrenergic receptors. Blood pressure response to phentolamine depends on the relative contri-butions of its vasodilating and cardiac stimulating effects.

At usual doses (and IV infusion rates ≥0.3 mg/min) vasodila-tion predominates, decreasing blood pressure and masking the in-otropic effect. Pulmonary vascular resistance and pulmonary arte-rial pressure are decreased. Cerebral blood flow is generally maintained.

Pharmacokinetics

Onset of Action: IV, 1–2 min; IM, 5–20 min.
Peak Effect: IV, 2 min; IM, <30 min.
Duration of Action: IV, 10–15 min; IM, 30–45 min.
Interaction/Toxicity: Use with epinephrine, ephedrine, do-butamine, or isoproterenol may cause paradoxical fall in blood pressure.

Guidelines/Precautions

1. Phentolamine-induced α-receptor blockade will potentiate the β_2-adrenergic vasodilation of epinephrine, ephedrine, do-butamine, or isoproterenol. Treat hypotension induced by phentolamine with norepinephrine.
2. Use with caution in patients with ischemic heart disease.

Principal Adverse Reactions

Cardiovascular: Hypotension, tachycardia, arrhythmias, myocar-dial infarction.
CNS: Dizziness, cerebrovascular spasm and occlusion.
GI: Nausea, vomiting, diarrhea.
Allergic: Flushing.

PHENYLEPHRINE HCL (NEO-SYNEPHRINE)

Use(s): Vasoconstrictor; treatment of hypotension, shock, su-praventricular tachyarrhythmias; prolongation of duration of local anesthetics.

Dosing: Hypotension during spinal or inhalation anesthesia: SC/
IM, 2–5 mg; IV, 50–100 μg (0.01% solution; dilute
0.1 mL 1% solution with 10 mL sterile water or NS
to give 100 μg/mL). Children, 1–2 μg/kg. Infusion,
0.15–0.75 μg/kg/min.

Paroxysmal supraventricular tachycardia: IV, 0.5–1
mg. Give rapidly within 20–30 sec. If cardiac rhythm
fails to convert within 60–90 sec, give an additional
2 mg IV slowly.

Vasoconstrictor for spinal anesthesia: 2–5 mg added to
anesthetic solution.

Vasoconstrictor for regional anesthesia: 1:20,000 dilution (1 mg diluted in 20 mL local anesthetic solution).

Nasal/topical: 2–3 drops/1–2 sprays of 0.25%–0.5%
solution. Use 0.125% solution in children <6 yr
old.

Elimination: Hepatic.

How Supplied: Injection, 1% solution (10 mg/mL); nasal solution, 0.125%, 0.16%, 0.2%, 0.5%, 0.25%, 1%.

Dilution for Infusion: 30 mg in 500 mL D_5W or NS solution
(60 μg/mL).

Pharmacology

Phenylephrine activates α-adrenergic receptors with minimal
β-activation. It produces intense peripheral vasoconstriction, increased systolic and diastolic blood pressures, and a reflex bradycardia that can result in decreased cardiac output. Renal, splanchnic, and cutaneous blood flows are reduced, but coronary blood
flow is increased because of increased work. Pulmonary artery
pressure is elevated. Reflex vagal effects can be used to slow the
heart rate in supraventricular tachyarrhythmias. Phenylephrine
decreases the rate of absorption of local anesthetics. It prolongs
the duration of anesthesia and decreases the risk of systemic toxicity.

Pharmacokinetics

Onset of Action: IV, almost immediate; IM/SC, 10–15 min.
Peak Effect: IV, 1 min.
Duration of Action: IV, 15–20 min; IM/SC, 30 min–2 hr.
Interaction/Toxicity: Pressor effects potentiated with oxytocics,
MAO inhibitors, guanethidine, bretylium, and other sympathomi-

metics; decreased or increased effects may occur with use of tricyclic antidepressants; sensitization of myocardium by volatile anesthetics may increase risk of arrhythmias with use of phenylephrine; extravasation may cause sloughing and necrosis.

Guidelines/Precautions

1. Use with extreme caution in elderly patients and patients with hyperthyroidism, bradycardia, partial heart block, or severe arteriosclerosis.
2. Use is not a substitute for the replacement of blood, plasma, fluids, and electrolytes, which should be restored promptly when loss has occurred.
3. Infuse into large veins to prevent extravasation. Treat any extravasation with local infiltration of phentolamine (5–10 mg in 10 mL NS solution) or sympathetic block.

Principal Adverse Reactions

Cardiovascular: Reflex bradycardia, arrhythmias, hypertension.
CNS: Headache, restlessness.

PHENYTOIN SODIUM (DILANTIN)

Use(s): Anticonvulsant, treatment of trigeminal neuralgia (tic douloureux), digitalis toxic arrhythmias, lidocaine-resistant ventricular arrhythmias, congenital prolonged QT-syndrome, and ventricular arrhythmias occurring after congenital heart surgery.
Dosing: Anticonvulsant: Loading IV/PO, 1 g (10–15 mg/kg) in 3 divided doses over 6 hr; maintenance IV and PO, 100 mg tid (Children, 5 mg/kg/day), do not exceed IV rate of 50 mg/min or 0.5–1.5 mg/kg/min in children; therapeutic range, 10–20 μg/mL.

Antiarrhythmic: IV, 1.5 mg/kg q5min until arrhythmia is controlled. Maximum dose, 10–15 mg/kg; PO, 200–400 mg once daily (2–4 mg/kg/day).
Elimination: Hepatic.
How Supplied: Injection, 50 mg/mL; capsules, 30 mg, 100 mg; capsules (extended release), 30 mg, 100 mg; tablets (chewable), 50 mg; oral suspension, 30 mg/5 mL, 125 mg/5 mL.

Pharmacology

Also called diphenylhydantoin, phenytoin is an anticonvulsant with primary site of action in the motor cortex. There it stabilizes the neuronal membranes and prevents the spread of activity through neuronal nets. Cellular electrical activity is stabilized by phenytoin by either preventing influx or enhancing efflux of sodium ions. It may be used for treatment of all kinds of epilepsy except petit mal epilepsy. It is also a class 1B antiarrhythmic. It decreases automaticity, duration of action potential, velocity of conduction, and effective refractory period of cardiac fibers.

Pharmacokinetics

Onset of Action: IV, few minutes.
Peak Effect: IV, 1–2 hr; PO, 4–12 hr.
Duration of Action: 10–15 hr (half-life).
Interaction/Toxicity: Serum level increased by diazepam, chloramphenicol, dicumarol, disulfiram, tolbutamide, salicylates, halothane, cimetidine, acute alcohol intake, sulfonamides, chlordiazepoxide; serum levels decreased by chronic alcohol abuse, reserpine, carbamazepine; oral absorption decreased by calcium-containing antacids; seizures precipitated with use of tricyclic antidepressants; decreases effects of corticosteroids, coumarin anticoagulants, quinidine, digitoxin, and furosemide; rapid IV administration may cause hypotension; may cause hyperglycemia, confusional states, SLE.

Guidelines/Precautions

1. Monitor serum blood levels to achieve optimal therapeutic effect.
2. Discontinue if rash occurs.
3. Because of its effect on ventricular automaticity, do not use IV phenytoin in sinus bradycardia, sinoatrial block, or second- and third-degree AV block or in patients with Adams-Stokes syndrome.
4. Use with caution in hypotension and severe myocardial insufficiency.
5. Abrupt withdrawal in epileptic patients may precipitate status epilepticus. Reduce dosage, discontinue, or substitute other anticonvulsant medications gradually.
6. Administration of phenytoin during pregnancy may result in

the fetal hydantoin syndrome. This may manifest as wide-set eyes, broad mandible, and finger deformities.

Principal Adverse Reactions

Cardiovascular: Hypotension, cardiovascular collapse, atrial and ventricular conduction depression, ventricular fibrillation.
CNS: Ataxia, confusion, dizziness, tremors, headaches, peripheral neuropathy.
GI: Nausea, vomiting, constipation.
Dermatologic: Stevens-Johnson syndrome, SLE, rash.
Hematologic: Thrombocytopenia, leukopenia, megaloblastic anemia.
Other: Hyperglycemia, gingival hyperplasia.

PHYSOSTIGMINE SALICYLATE (ANTILIRIUM)

Use(s): Reversal of drug-induced (anticholinergic) CNS effects, topical treatment of glaucoma.
Dosing: Anticholinergic reversal: IV/IM, 0.5–2 mg (10–30 μg/kg) rate of 1 mg/min, repeat at intervals of 10–30 min if desired patient response is not obtained.
Elimination: Plasma esterases.
How Supplied: Injection, 1 mg/mL.

Pharmacology

This tertiary amine anticholinesterase agent effectively increases the concentration of acetylcholine at sites of cholinergic transmission and facilitates the transmission of impulses across the neuromuscular junction. Unlike neostigmine, physostigmine penetrates the blood brain barrier. It reverses the central anticholinergic syndrome (anxiety, confusion, seizures) and peripheral anticholinergia (hyperpyrexia, vasodilation, urinary retention) associated with anticholinergic drugs (e.g., atropine, scopolamine, tricyclic antidepressants). Can also reverse the sedative effects of benzodiazepines (e.g., diazepam), phenothiazines, and the ventilatory depressant effects of opioids. It may reduce postoperative somnolence following use of a volatile anesthetic.

Pharmacokinetics

Onset of Action: IV/IM, 3–8 min.
Peak Effect: IV/IM, 5–10 min.
Duration of Action: IV/IM, 30 min–5 hr.
Interaction/Toxicity: Overdosage may cause cholinergic crisis (bronchoconstriction, excessive salivation and sweating, bradycardia, skeletal muscle paresis or paralysis, hallucinations, seizures).

Guidelines/Precautions

1. Because of its potential for producing serious adverse effects (e.g., seizures), routine use of physostigmine as an antidote for overdosage of anticholinergic drugs is controversial.
2. High doses may cause tremors, ataxia, muscle fasciculations, and ultimately a depolarization block.
3. Rapid IV administration can cause bradycardia, hypersalivation, leading to respiratory problems or possibly seizures.
4. Treatment of cholinergic crisis includes mechanical ventilation with repeated bronchial aspiration and IV atropine, 2–4 mg q3–10 min, until control of muscarinic symptoms is achieved or signs of atropine overdosage appear. IV pralidoxime (15 mg/kg over 2 min) may be useful in counteracting the ganglionic and skeletal muscle effects of physostigmine.
5. Use with caution in patients with epilepsy, parkinsonian syndrome, or bradycardia.
6. Do not use in the presence of asthma, diabetes, mechanical obstruction of the intestine or urogenital tract, and in patients receiving choline esters or depolarizing muscle relaxants.

Principal Adverse Reactions

Cardiovascular: Bradycardia.
Pulmonary: Bronchospasm, dyspnea, respiratory paralysis.
CNS: Seizures.
GI: Salivation, nausea, vomiting.
Eye: Miosis.

PHYTONADIONE–VITAMIN K (AQUAMEPHYTON, KONAKION)

Use(s): Treatment of hypoprothrombinemia, prophylaxis and treatment of hemorrhagic diseases of the newborn; reversal of effects of oral anticoagulants.

Dosing: Hemorrhagic diseases of the newborn: Prophylaxis (newborn), IM/SC, 0.5–1 mg within 1 hr after birth; (mother), IM, 1–5 mg 12–24 hr before delivery; treatment (newborn), IM/SC, 1 mg (higher doses may be necessary if the mother has received anticoagulants); failure to respond may indicate another diagnosis or coagulation disorder.

Hypoprothrombinemia: Adults: IV/IM/SC/PO: 2.5–25 mg. IV rate, 1 mg/min.

Elimination: Hepatic.

How Supplied: Injection, 10 mg/mL; tablets, 5 mg.

Pharmacology

An aqueous dispersion of vitamin K_1, which is necessary for the hepatic synthesis of prothrombin (factor II), proconvertin (factor VII), plasma thromboplastin component (factor IX), and Stuart factor (factor X). The mechanism by which vitamin K promotes formation of these clotting factors in the liver is not known. It is ineffective in severe hypoprothrombinemia and against heparin-induced anticoagulation. Give whole blood or component therapy concurrently when bleeding is severe.

Pharmacokinetics

Onset of Action: IV/IM/SC, 1–2 hr; PO, 6–12 hr.
Peak Effect: IV/IM/SC, 3–6 hr (normal PT within 12–14 hr).
Duration of Action: Varies.
Interaction/Toxicity: Pharmacologic antagonist to coumarin and indandione derivatives; decreased absorption with concurrent oral administration of cholestyramine or mineral oil.

Guidelines/Precautions

1. Slow onset of action. Fresh plasma or blood transfusion may be required for severe blood loss or lack of response to vitamin K.

2. Periodic monitoring of PT. Overzealous therapy with vitamin K may restore conditions that originally permitted thromboembolic phenomena.
3. Failure to respond to vitamin K may indicate the presence of coagulation defect or that the condition being treated is unresponsive to vitamin K.
4. Anaphylactic shock and death after IV injection. Restrict IV route to situations where other routes of administration are not available.

Principal Adverse Reactions

Cardiovascular: Cardiac arrest, hypotension.
Pulmonary: Respiratory arrest, dyspnea.
CNS: Dizziness.
Dermatologic: Local hemorrhage at injection site.
Allergic: Shock, anaphylaxis (with IV injection).
Hematologic: Hyperbilirubinemia at injection site.

PIPECURONIUM BROMIDE (ARDUAN)

Use(s): Nondepolarizing muscle relaxant.
Dosing: IV (paralyzing), 0.07–0.085 mg/kg.
　　　　　　Pretreatment and maintenance, 0.01–0.015 mg/kg.
Elimination: Renal.
How Supplied: Powder for injection: 10 mg.

Pharmacology

This long-acting nondepolarizing neuromuscular blocking agent is a piperazinium derivative. It acts by competing for cholinergic receptors at the motor end plate. The time of onset and duration are similar to those of pancuronium at comparable doses. The drug has no clinically significant hemodynamic effects. Histamine release rarely occurs.

Pharmacokinetics

Onset of Action: <3 min.
Peak Effect: 3–5 min.
Duration of Action: 45–120 min.

Interaction/Toxicity: Potentiated by prior administration of succinylcholine, volatile anesthetics, aminoglycoside antibiotics, local anesthetics, loop diuretics, magnesium, lithium, phenytoin, ganglionic blocking drugs, hypothermia, hypokalemia, respiratory acidosis; recurrent paralysis with quinidine, enhanced neuromuscular blockade in patients with myasthenia gravis or inadequate adrenocortical function; effects antagonized by anticholinesterase inhibitors such as neostigmine, edrophonium, pyridostigmine; increased resistance or reversal of effects with use of theophylline and in patients with burn injury and paresis.

Guidelines/Precautions

1. Monitor response with peripheral nerve stimulator to minimize risk of overdosage.
2. Reverse effects with anticholinesterases such as pyridostigmine bromide, neostigmine, or edrophonium in conjunction with atropine or glycopyrrolate.
3. Pretreatment doses may induce a degree of neuromuscular blockade sufficient to cause hypoventilation in some patients.

Principal Adverse Reactions

Cardiovascular: Hypotension, hypertension, bradycardia, myocardial infarction.
Pulmonary: Hypoventilation, apnea.
CNS: Depression.
GU: Anuria.
Dermatologic: Rash, urticaria.
Musculoskeletal: Inadequate block, prolonged block.
Metabolic: Hypoglycemia, hyperkalemia, increased creatinine.

POTASSIUM CHLORIDE (POTASSIUM CHLORIDE)

Use(s): Electrolyte replacement, treatment of hypokalemia, treatment of cardiac arrhythmias associated with digitalis toxicity and hypokalemia.
Dosing: IV: 10–20 mEq/hr. Dilute before use. Maximum concentration, 40 mEq/L of IV fluid. In critical condi-

tions, with close ECG monitoring, higher rates
(20–40 mEq/hr) and concentrations (60–80 mEq/L)
may be administered. Maximum 24-hr dose, 200
mEq with serum potassium >2.5 mEq/L and 400
mEq with serum potassium <2.5 mEq/L. Children:
IV infusion up to 3 mEq/kg, or 40 mEq/m^2/day.
Monitoring of the ECG and plasma potassium concentrations is essential during IV administration of
potassium. Do not administer undiluted potassium.
Potassium preparations must be diluted with suitable
large-volume parenteral solutions (preferably NS),
mixed well, and given by slow IV infusion.

> PO: 20–100 mEq daily (2–4 divided doses). Maxi-
> mum daily requirements for infants, 2–3 mEq/kg,
> or 40 mEq/m^2.

Elimination: Renal.
How Supplied: Injection: 20 mEq/10 mL, 30 mEq/15 mL, 40
mEq/20 mL, 60 mEq/30 mL, 400 mEq/200 mL; capsules (extended release): 8 mEq, 10 mEq, 20 mEq; for solution: 15 mEq/
packet, 20 mEq/packet, 25 mEq/packet; for suspension (extended
release): 20 mEq/packet; solution: 6.7 mEq/5 mL, 10.0 mEq/5
mL, 13.3 mEq/5 mL, 10 mEq/15 mL, 10 mEq/15 mL, 15 mEq/15
mL, 20 mEq/15 mL, 30 mEq/15 mL, 40 mEq/15 mL.

Pharmacology

Potassium is the major cation of intracellular fluid. It is essential
for maintenance of intracellular tonicity and acid-base balance.
Potassium is an important activator in many enzymatic reactions
and is essential in a number of physiologic processes, including
transmission of nerve impulses; contraction of cardiac, skeletal,
and smooth muscles; gastric secretion; renal function; tissue synthesis; and carbohydrate metabolism. After absorption, potassium
first enters the extracellular fluid and is then actively transported
into the cells, where its concentration is up to 40 times that out-
side the cell. Dextrose, insulin, and oxygen facilitate movement
of potassium into cells. In healthy adults, plasma potassium concentrations generally range from 3.5–5 mEq/L. Plasma concentrations up to 7.7 mEq/L may be normal in neonates. Plasma potassium concentrations, however, are not necessarily accurate
indications of cellular potassium concentrations; cellular deficits

can occur without decreases in plasma potassium concentrations, and hypokalemia may occur without substantial depletion of cellular potassium. Changes in extracellular fluid pH produce reciprocal effects on plasma potassium concentrations. A change of 0.1 unit in plasma pH may produce an inverse change of 0.6 mEq/L in plasma potassium concentration. Potassium concentrations in gastric and intestinal secretions are higher than plasma concentrations.

Pharmacokinetics

Onset of Action: IV: Immediate.
Peak Effect: IV: Varies.
Duration of Action: IV: Varies.
Interaction/Toxicity: Severe or life-threatening hyperkalemia may occur with concomitant administration of ACE inhibitors, potassium-sparing diuretics, and salt substitutes; GI toxicity is enhanced by anticholinergic drugs (e.g., atropine, glycopyrrolate), which delay gastric emptying.

Guidelines/Precautions

1. Concentrated potassium solutions are for IV admixtures only; do not use undiluted. Direct injection may be instantaneously fatal.
2. Do not infuse rapidly. Base therapy on close medical supervision with continuous or serial ECG and serum potassium determinations. Plasma levels are not necessarily indicative of tissue levels.
3. Use with caution in the presence of cardiac disease, particularly in digitalized patients (with bradyarrhythmias and potassium levels >3 mEq/liter) or in the presence of renal disease, metabolic acidosis, Addison's disease, prolonged or severe diarrhea, familial periodic paralysis, hypoadrenalism, hyponatremia, and myotonia congenita.
4. Hypokalemia associated with metabolic acidosis should be treated with an alkalinizing potassium salt (e.g., potassium bicarbonate, citrate, gluconate, or acetate).
5. In states of dehydration and shock, do not replenish potassium until hydration and diuresis are established.
6. Intestinal and gastric ulceration and bleeding have occurred with extended-release potassium chloride preparations. These

dosage forms should be reserved for patients who cannot tolerate or refuse to take liquid or effervescent preparations. Do not use solid oral dosage forms in patients in whom there is a structural, pathologic (e.g., diabetic gastroparesis), and/or pharmacologic (e.g., induced by anticholinergics) cause for arrest or delay in passage of the dosage form through the GI tract; an oral liquid preparation should be used in these patients.

7. High plasma concentrations of potassium may cause death through cardiac depression, arrhythmia, or arrest.

8. Signs and symptoms of hyperkalemia include paresthesia of extremities; flaccid paralysis; muscle or respiratory paralysis; areflexia; weakness; listlessness; mental confusion; weakness and heaviness of legs; hypotension; cardiac arrhythmias; heart block; ECG abnormalities such as tall peaked T waves, depression of the ST segment, disappearance of P waves, prolongation of the QT interval, spreading and slurring of the QRS complex with development of a biphasic curve and cardiac arrest.

9. Treat hyperkalemia by immediate termination of potassium administration. Monitor ECG. Infusion of combined glucose and insulin in a ratio of 3 g glucose to 1 unit regular insulin may be administered to shift potassium into cells. Administer sodium bicarbonate (50–100 mEq IV) to reverse acidosis and also produce an intracellular shift. Give 10–100 mL calcium gluconate or calcium chloride 10% to reverse ECG changes. To remove potassium from the body, use sodium polysterene sulfonate resin or hemodialysis or peritoneal dialysis. In digitalized patients, too rapid lowering of serum potassium levels can cause digitalis toxicity.

10. Treat extravasation by discontinuing IV administration at that site and local infiltration with 1% procaine HCl and hyaluronidase.

Principal Adverse Reactions

Cardiovascular: Arrhythmias, cardiac arrest.
CNS: Lethargy, coma.
GI: Nausea, vomiting, abdominal pain, esophageal/small bowel ulceration.

Dermatologic: Phlebitis at injection site, sloughing, necrosis, abscess formation.
Metabolic: Hyperkalemia.

PRILOCAINE HCL (CITANEST)*

Use(s): Regional anesthesia.
Dosing: IV regional block: Upper extremities, 200–250 mg
(40–50 mL 0.5% solution); lower extremities,
250–300 mg (100–120 mL 0.25% solution); do not
add epinephrine; rate of onset and potency of local
anesthetic action may be enhanced by carbonation
(add 5 mL 8.4% sodium bicarbonate with 40 mL
0.5% prilocaine); do not use if there is precipitation.
Topical: 0.6–3 mg/kg (2%–4% solution).
Infiltration/peripheral nerve block: 0.5–6 mg/kg
(0.5%–2% solution).
Brachial plexus block: 300–600 mg (30–40 mL of
1%–1.5% solution). Children, 0.2–0.33 mL/kg.
Epidural: 200–300 mg (1%–2% solution). Maximum
safe dose: 6 mg/kg without epinephrine; 9 mg/kg with
epinephrine 1:200,000. Solutions containing preservatives should not be used for epidural block.
Elimination: Hepatic, pulmonary.
How Supplied: Injection, 4% with or without epinephrine
1:200,000.

Pharmacology

This amide local anesthetic stabilizes the neuronal membrane and
prevents the initiation and transmission of impulses. Equipotent to
lidocaine but longer in duration; it is less toxic and undergoes
rapid hepatic metabolism to orthotoluidine, which oxidizes hemoglobin to methemoglobin. When the dose of prilocaine exceeds
600 mg, there may be sufficient methemoglobin to cause the patient
to appear cyanotic, and oxygen-carrying capacity is reduced. The

*For additional precautions, see Bupivacaine, Guidelines/Precautions, items 8 to
10, p 20.

unique ability to cause dose-related methemoglobinemia limits its clinical usefulness, with the exception of IV regional anesthesia.

Pharmacokinetics

Onset of Action: Infiltration, 1–2 min; epidural, 5–15 min.
Peak Effect: Infiltration/epidural: <30 min.
Duration of Action: Infiltration: 0.5–1.5 hr without epinephrine, 2–6 hr with epinephrine.
Epidural: 1–3 hr; prolonged with epinephrine.
Interaction/Toxicity: Methemoglobinemia at high doses (>600 mg); reduced clearance with coadministration of β-blockers, cimetidine; toxic drug concentrations may result in seizures, respiratory depression, cardiovascular collapse; duration of local or regional anesthesia prolonged by vasoconstrictor agents, e.g., epinephrine.

Guidelines/Precautions

1. Treat methemoglobinemia with methylene blue (1–2 mg/kg injected over 5 min).
2. Use with caution in patients with hypovolemia, severe CHF, shock, and all forms of heart block.
3. Contraindicated in infants <6 mo old (low dose may cause methemoglobinemia) and in patients with hypersensitivity to amide-type local anesthetics.
4. In IV regional blocks, deflate the cuff after 40 min and no <20 min. Between 20 and 40 min, the cuff can be deflated, reinflated immediately, and finally deflated after 1 min to reduce the sudden absorption of anesthetic into the systemic circulation.

Principal Adverse Reactions

Cardiovascular: Hypotension, arrhythmia, collapse.
Pulmonary: Respiratory depression, paralysis.
CNS: Seizures, tinnitus, blurred vision.
Hematologic: Methemoglobinemia.
Allergic: Urticaria, anaphylactoid reactions.
Epidural/Caudal: High spinal, urinary retention, lower extremity weakness and paralysis, loss of sphincter control, headache, backache, cranial nerve palsies, slowing of labor.

PROCAINAMIDE HCL (PROCAN SR, PRONESTYL)

Use(s): Arrhythmia control in malignant hyperthermia; treatment of lidocaine-resistant ventricular arrhythmias, atrial fibrillation, or paroxysmal atrial tachycardia.

Dosing: Loading slow IV push: 100 mg every 5 min (maximum, 1 g). Do not exceed 50 mg/min. (Children: 3–6 mg/kg given over 5 min.) Dilute 1000 mg in 50 mL D_5W or

    IM, 100–500 mg, or

    PO, 1.25 g, then 750 mg 1 hr later if there are no changes in ECG.

    Maintenance: Infusion, 2–6 mg/min (children: 0.02–0.08 mg/kg/min) or PO, 0.5–1 g q3–6h (q6h with SR tablets). Children: 40–60 mg/kg/day in 4 divided doses.

    Therapeutic level: 4–12 µg/mL.

Elimination: Hepatic (acetylation).

How Supplied: Injection: 100 mg/mL, 500 mg/mL; tablets: 250 mg, 375 mg, 500 mg; tablets (SR): 250 mg, 500 mg, 750 mg, 1000 mg (do not use SR tablets for initial oral therapy); capsules, 250 mg, 375 mg, 500 mg.

Dilution for Infusion: 2 g in 500 mL D_5W (4 mg/mL).

Pharmacology

Procainamide, like quinidine and disopyramide, is a class 1A antiarrhythmic (membrane stabilizer). It increases the effective refractory period and reduces impulse conduction velocity in the atria, His-Purkinje fibers, and ventricular muscle. It has a variable effect on AV conduction, with a direct slowing action and weaker vagolytic effect on the AV node. Direct myocardial depression at high plasma levels (>8 µg/mL). Antiarrhythmic effect seen at plasma levels of 4–12 µg/mL. Procainamide is an effective alternative for acute treatment of lidocaine-resistant ventricular arrhythmias.

Pharmacokinetics

Onset of Action: IV: immediate; IM: 10–30 min.
Peak Effect: IV: 5–15 min, IM: 15–60 min.

Duration of Action: 2.5 hr (half-life in fast acetylators); 5 hr (half-life in slow acetylators).

Interaction/Toxicity: Hypotension with rapid IV administration and potentiated by use of other antiarrythmics; may cause myocardial depression, ventricular arrhythmias at high plasma levels exaggerated by hyperkalemia; ventricular asystole or fibrillation in the presence of heart block associated with digitalis toxicity; SLE-like syndrome; potentiates effect of both nondepolarizing and depolarizing muscle relaxants; increased serum levels with concomitant administration of cimetidine and ranitidine.

Guidelines/Precautions

1. Reduce doses in the presence of CHF and renal failure.
2. Contraindicated in complete heart block, torsades de Pointes, SLE.
3. Patients with atrial flutter or fibrillation should be cardioverted or heart rate controlled, e.g., with digitalis, β-blockers, calcium channel blockers, before procainamide administration to avoid enhancement of AV conduction and intolerable ventricular rate acceleration.
4. Use cautiously in first-degree heart block and arrhythmias associated with digitalis intoxication.
5. Periodic monitoring of plasma levels, vital signs, ECG (QRS widening of >25% may signify overdosage).

Principal Adverse Reactions

Cardiovascular: Hypotension, heart block, arrhythmias.
CNS: Seizures, confusion, depression, psychosis.
GI: Anorexia, nausea, vomiting, diarrhea (usually with large oral doses).
Dermatologic: SLE, urticaria, pruritus.
Hematologic: Thrombocytopenia, neutropenia, hemolytic anemia, agranulocytosis.
Allergic: Angioneurotic edema, eosinophilia.
Others: Fever, chills.

PROCAINE HCL (NOVOCAIN)*

Use(s): Regional anesthesia.
Dosing: Infiltration, <500 mg (0.5%–2% solution).
           Epidural, <500 mg (1%–2% solution) (solutions containing preservatives should not be used for epidural or spinal block).
           Spinal, 50–200 mg (10% solution with glucose 5%).
           Maximum safe dose, 500 mg (without epinephrine), 1000 mg (with epinephrine).
Elimination: Plasma pseudocholinesterase.
How Supplied: Injection, 1%, 2%; spinal, 10% (hyperbaric solution).

Pharmacology

Procaine is a benzoic acid ester local anesthetic. It stabilizes the neuronal membrane and prevents the initiation and transmission of impulses. It possesses vasodilator activity and is ineffective as a surface anesthetic. It has a rapid onset of action and a relatively short duration, depending on the anesthetic technique, the type of block, concentration, and the individual patient. Vasoconstrictor drugs may be added to the procaine solution to delay systemic absorption and prolong the duration of action.

Pharmacokinetics

Onset of Action: Infiltration/spinal, 2–5 min; epidural, 5–25 min.
Peak Effect: Infiltration/epidural/spinal, <30 min.
Duration of Action: Infiltration, 0.25–0.5 hr (without epinephrine), 0.5–1.5 hr with epinephrine; epidural/spinal, 0.5–1.5 hr (prolonged with epinephrine).
Interaction/Toxicity: Prolongs the effect of succinylcholine; metabolite (PABA) inhibits action of sulfonamides; toxicity enhanced by anticholinesterases (which inhibits degradation); high plasma levels may cause seizures, respiratory arrest, cardiovascular collapse; duration of local or regional anesthesia prolonged by vasoconstrictor agents, e.g., epinephrine.

*For additional precautions, see Bupivacaine, Guidelines/Precautions, items 8 to 10, p 20.

Guidelines/Precautions

1. Use with caution in patients with severe disturbances of cardiac rhythm, shock, or heart block.
2. Reduce doses for spinal anesthesia in obstetric, elderly, hypovolemic, and high-risk patients and those with increased intra-abdominal pressure.
3. Contraindicated in patients with hypersensitivity to procaine or ester-type local anesthetics.

Principal Adverse Reactions

Cardiovascular: Hypotension, bradycardia, arrhythmias, heart block.
Pulmonary: Respiratory depression, arrest.
CNS: Tinnitus, seizures, dizziness, restlessness, loss of hearing, euphoria, diplopia, postspinal headache, arachnoiditis, palsies.
Allergic: Urticaria, pruritus, angioneurotic edema.
Epidural/Caudal/Spinal: High spinal, loss of bladder and bowel control, permanent motor, sensory, autonomic (sphincter control), deficit of lower segments.

PROCHLORPERAZINE (COMPAZINE)

Use(s): Antiemetic; antipsychotic.
Dosing: Antiemetic: PO, 5–10 mg tid or qid; rectal, 25 mg bid; IV/IM, 5–10 mg (at 5 mg/mL/min). Do not administer SC because of local irritation.
Elimination: Hepatic.
How Supplied: Tablets: 5 mg, 10 mg, 25 mg; capsules (extended release), 10 mg, 15 mg, 30 mg; suppositories, 2.5 mg, 5 mg, 25 mg; injection, 5 mg/mL.

Pharmacology

Prochlorperazine is a piperazine phenothiazine. Its antipsychotic activity is thought to result from the drug's central antidopaminergic actions. Its antiemetic action is mediated via the chemoreceptor trigger zone of the medulla. It produces α-adrenergic blockade, which may result in hypotension. Prochlorperazine interferes with central thermoregulatory mechanisms and may produce tardive dyskinesia and extrapyramidal symptoms secondary to blockade of dopaminergic receptors in the basal ganglia.

Pharmacokinetics

Onset of Action: IV, few minutes; IM, 10–20 min; PO, 30–40 min; rectal, 60 min.
Peak Effect: IV/IM/PO: 15–30 min.
Duration of Action: IV/IM/PO/rectal, 3–4 hr; PO, extended release, 10–12 hr.
Interaction/Toxicity: Potentiates CNS and circulatory depressant effects of alcohol, opioids, barbiturates, antihistamines; diminishes effects of oral anticoagulants; counteracts antihypertensive effect of propranolol; decreases metabolism of phenytoin; lowers seizure threshold and increases dosage requirements for anticonvulsant agents; acute encephalopathic syndrome may occur in the presence of high serum lithium levels; hypotension from rapid IV injection; mephentermine, epinephrine, thiazide diuretics potentiate prochlorperazine-induced hypotension; may induce extrapyramidal symptoms, neuroleptic malignant syndrome.

Guidelines/Precautions

1. Extrapyramidal reactions may consist of dystonic reactions, feelings of motor restlessness (akathisia), and parkinsonian signs and symptoms. Dystonic reactions occur more frequently in children, especially those with acute infections, whereas parkinsonian symptoms predominate in geriatric patients. Therapy should include discontinuation or reduction in dosage and treatment with an anticholinergic antiparkinsonian agent (e.g., benztropine, trihexyphenidyl) or diphenhydramine (IV/PO, 25 mg). Maintenance of an adequate airway should be instituted if necessary.
2. Use cautiously in geriatric patients; patients with glaucoma, prostatic hypertrophy, or seizure disorders; and children with acute illnesses (e.g., chickenpox, measles).
3. Do not use in pediatric surgery.
4. Neuroleptic malignant syndrome (hyperpyrexia, tachycardia, muscle rigidity) should be managed by immediate discontinuation of prochlorperazine and symptomatic and supportive treatment, including correction of fluid and electrolyte imbalances, administration of dantrolene, cooling of the patient,

maintenance of renal function, management of cardiovascular instability, and prevention of respiratory complications.
5. Possesses little or no antimotion sickness activity.
6. Do not crush or chew SR capsules.
7. Do not use epinephrine to treat prochlorperazine-induced hypotension. Phenothiazines cause a reversal of the vasopressor effects of epinephrine, and a further lowering of blood pressure. Treat the drug-induced hypotension with norepinephrine or phenylephrine.

Principal Adverse Reactions

Cardiovascular: Hypotension, hypertension.
Pulmonary: Bronchospasm, laryngeal edema.
CNS: Drowsiness, dizziness, extrapyramidal reactions, tardive dyskinesia.
GI/Hepatic: Cholestatic jaundice, nausea, vomiting.
Endocrine: Gynecomastia, amenorrhea, hyperglycemia.
Allergic: Angioneurotic edema, anaphylactoid reactions.

PROMETHAZINE HCL (PHENERGAN)

Use(s): Antiemetic, premedication, adjunct to analgesics for control of postoperative pain.
Dosing: IV/deep IM/PO/rectal, 12.5–50 mg (do not give SC).
Elimination: Hepatic.
How Supplied: Injection: 25 mg/mL, 50 mg/mL; tablets/suppositories: 12.5 mg, 25 mg, 50 mg; oral solution: 6.25 mg/5 mL, 25 mg/5 mL.

Pharmacology

This phenothiazine derivative does not possess neuroleptic or antipsychotic activity in typical standard doses. It is a good histamine H_1 receptor antagonist with sedative, antiemetic, anticholinergic, and antimotion sickness effects. Competitively antagonizes in varying degrees most but not all of the pharmacologic effects of histamine mediated at H_1 receptors. Not effective in the treatment of bronchial asthma, allergic reactions, or angioedema in which chemical mediators other than histamine are responsible for the symptoms.

Pharmacokinetics

Onset of Action: IV, 2–5 min; IM/PO/rectal, 15–30 min.
Peak Effect: IV/IM/PO/rectal, <2 hr.
Duration of Action: IV/IM/PO/rectal, 2–8 hr.
Interaction/Toxicity: Potentiates CNS and circulatory depressant effect of alcohol, sedative hypnotics, including barbiturates, volatile anesthetics, tranquilizers; intra-arterial or SC injection may result in necrosis and gangrene; may reverse vasopressor effect of epinephrine; extrapyramidal reactions at high doses and with concomitant use of MAO inhibitors.

Guidelines/Precautions

1. Extrapyramidal reactions may consist of dystonic reactions, feelings of motor restlessness (akathisia), and parkinsonian signs and symptoms. Dystonic reactions occur more frequently in children, especially those with acute infections, whereas parkinsonian symptoms predominate in geriatric patients. Therapy should include discontinuation or reduction in dosage and treatment with an anticholinergic antiparkinsonian agent (e.g., benztropine, trihexyphenidyl) or with diphenhydramine (IV/PO, 25 mg). Maintenance of an adequate airway should be instituted if necessary.
2. Use with caution in patients with cardiovascular disease, liver dysfunction, asthmatic attack, narrow-angle glaucoma, bone marrow depression, prostatic hypertrophy, stenosing peptic ulcer; pyloroduodenal and bladder neck obstruction.
3. Use with caution, if at all, in children.
4. Produces a high degree of drowsiness and sedation at clinically effective doses.
5. Do not use epinephrine to treat promethazine-induced hypotension. Phenothiazines cause a reversal of the vasopressor effects of epinephrine and a further lowering of blood pressure. Treat the drug-induced hypotension with norepinephrine or phenylephrine.

Principal Adverse Reactions

Cardiovascular: Hypotension, bradycardia, tachycardia, extrasystoles.
Pulmonary: Bronchospasm, nasal stuffiness.
CNS: Drowsiness, sedation, dizziness, confusion, tremors.

GI: Nausea, vomiting.
Hematologic: Leukopenia, agranulocytosis, thrombocytopenia.

PROPOFOL (DIPRIVAN)

Use(s): Induction agent, maintenance of anesthesia.
Dosing: IV (bolus), 25–50 mg; induction, 2–2.5 mg/kg. (40 mg q10sec until onset of induction); infusion, 100–200 μg/kg/min.
Elimination: Hepatic, extrahepatic.
How Supplied: Injection: 10 mg/mL.
Dilution for Infusion: Use undiluted or dilute with D_5W to concentration ≥2 mg/mL. Discard after use. There is no preservative.

Pharmacology

Propofol is a diisopropylphenol, IV hypnotic agent that produces rapid induction of anesthesia with minimal excitatory activity (e.g., myoclonus). It undergoes extensive distribution and rapid elimination. Induction doses are associated with apnea and hypotension secondary to direct myocardial depression and a decrease in systemic vascular resistance with minimal change in heart rate. The drug obtunds the hemodynamic response to laryngoscopy and intubation. Propofol does not have any analgesic effect, but unlike barbiturates it is not antianalgesic. Compared with thiopental, recovery is more rapid, and there is less nausea and vomiting. Histamine release may occur.

Pharmacokinetics

Onset of Action: Within 40 sec.
Peak Effect: 1 min.
Duration of Action: 5–10 min.
Interaction/Toxicity: Potentiates CNS and circulatory depressant effects of narcotics, sedative hypnotics, volatile anesthetics; pain on injection into small vein.

Guidelines/Precautions

1. Reduce doses in elderly, hypovolemic, high-risk patients, and with concomitant use of narcotics and sedative hypnotics.
2. Minimize pain by injecting in a large vein and/or mixing IV

lidocaine (0.1 mg/kg) with the induction dose of propofol.
3. Contraindicated in patients allergic to eggs.

Principal Adverse Reactions

Cardiovascular: Hypotension, arrhythmia, tachycardia, bradycardia, hypertension.
Pulmonary: Respiratory depression, apnea, hiccups, bronchospasm, laryngospasm.
CNS: Headache, dizziness, euphoria, confusion, clonic myoclonic movement.
GI: Nausea, vomiting, abdominal cramps.
Local: Burning, stinging, pain at the injection site.
Allergic: Erythema, urticaria, pruritus.
Other: Fever.

PROPRANOLOL HCL (INDERAL)

Use(s): Antihypertensive, antianginal, antiarrhythmic (supraventricular and ventricular arrhythmias), treatment of acute myocardial infarction, migraine prophylaxis, symptomatic treatment of thyrotoxicosis, pheochromocytoma, and tremors.
Dosing: Hypertension: IV, 0.5–3.0 mg (10–30 μg/kg) q2min to maximum of 6–10 mg; PO, 20–80 mg in single or divided doses; therapeutic concentration, 50–100 ng/mL.

Arrhythmia: PO, 10–30 mg tid or qid; IV, 0.5–3.0 mg (10–30 μg/kg) q2min to maximum of 6–10 mg.

Angina: PO, 80–320 mg in single or divided doses at weekly intervals.

Acute myocardial infarction: IV, 1–3 mg (do not exceed 1 mg/min to avoid lowering the blood pressure and causing cardiac standstill. If necessary, give a second dose after 2 min) then PO, 180–240 mg/day in 3 or 4 divided doses.

Migraine prophylaxis: PO, 80 mg once daily.
Elimination: Hepatic.
How Supplied: Injection: 1 mg/mL; tablets: 10 mg, 20 mg, 40 mg, 60 mg, 80 mg, 90 mg; Capsules (extended release): 60 mg, 80 mg, 120 mg, 160 mg; oral solution: 20 mg/5 mL, 40 mg/5 mL, 80 mg/5 mL.

Pharmacology

Propranolol is a nonselective β-adrenergic receptor antagonist without intrinsic sympathomimetic activity. The degree of reduction of β-actions depends on the ongoing β-activity at the time of administration. Thus, decreases in heart rate and cardiac output (β₁-receptor blockade) are greater in the presence of increased sympathetic nervous system activity. Blockade of β₂-receptors increases peripheral and coronary vascular resistance. Reduced cardiac work is the basis for use of the drug after myocardial infarction and in the treatment of angina. Propranolol depresses automaticity and conduction velocity in cardiac muscle.

Pharmacokinetics

Onset of Action: IV, <2 min; PO, <30 min.
Peak Effect: IV, within 1 min; PO, varies.
Duration of Action: IV, $1-6$ hr; PO, $6-12$ hr.
Interaction/Toxicity: Potentiates myocardial depression of inhaled and injected anesthetics; additive effects with catecholamine-depleting drugs (e.g., reserpine), calcium channel blockers; antagonizes cardiac-stimulating and bronchodilating effects of sympathomimetics; potentiates vasoconstrictive effects of epinephrine; increased serum levels with concomitant use of chlorpromazine, cimetidine; decreased serum levels with enzyme inducers (e.g., phenytoin, phenobarbital, rifampin); decreases clearance of theophylline, lidocaine; potentiates effects of succinylcholine, tubocurarine, digoxin; produces hypoglycemia, prolongs the hypoglycemic effect of insulin, and may mask symptoms of hypoglycemia (e.g., tachycardia); may unmask direct negative inotropic effects of ketamine.

Guidelines/Precautions

1. Contraindicated in cardiogenic shock, sinus bradycardia, and greater than first-degree block, bronchial asthma, CHF unless the failure is secondary to a tachyarrhythmia treatable with propranolol.
2. Use with caution in patients with diabetes and nonallergic bronchospastic disease (e.g., bronchitis).
3. Excessive myocardial depression may be treated with IV atropine ($1-2$ mg), IV isoproterenol ($0.02-0.15$ µg/kg/min), or a transvenous cardiac pacemaker.
4. Increased risk of ischemia or infarction in patients with coronary artery disease if drug is withdrawn abruptly.

5. Concomitant epinephrine use may cause rapid BP increase and pulse rate decrease.

Principal Adverse Reactions

Cardiovascular: Bradycardia, hypotension, CHF, AV block.
Pulmonary: Bronchospasm.
CNS: Depression, disorientation, dizziness, memory loss.
GI: Nausea, vomiting, mesenteric thrombosis.
Hematologic: Agranulocytosis, thrombocytopenic purpura, non-thrombocytopenic purpura.

PROSTAGLANDIN E_1—ALPROSTADIL (PROSTIN VR)

Use(s): Maintain patency of patent ductus arteriosus, treatment of severe pulmonary hypertension with right-sided heart failure.
Dosing: IV, 0.05–0.4 μg/kg/min (titrate to lowest effective dose).
Elimination: Pulmonary (oxidation).
How Supplied: Injection, 500 μg/mL.
Dilution for Infusion: 500 μg in 250 mL D_5W or NS solution (2 μg/mL).

Pharmacology

Prostaglandin E_1 (PGE_1) relaxes smooth muscle of the ductus arteriosus. This is beneficial in infants who have congenital defects that restrict the pulmonary or systemic blood flow and who depend on a patent ductus arteriosus for adequate blood oxygenation. PGE_1 produces vasodilation and reduces blood pressure, resulting in a reflex increase in cardiac output and heart rate. In infants with restricted systemic blood flow, it increases the systemic blood pressure and decreases the ratio of pulmonary artery pressure to aortic pressure. Infants who respond best are less than 4 days old with low pretreatment Po_2 (<40 mm Hg).
In treatment of severe pulmonary hypertension with right-sided heart failure, PGE_1 may be infused into the right atrium, from which point it proceeds directly to the pulmonary artery and attenuates pulmonary vasoconstriction. Because of lung metabolism, relatively less of the drug passes on to the systemic vasculature. The systemic vasodilation is reversed by infusing norepinephrine into the left atrium simultaneously.

Pharmacokinetics

Onset of Action: Cyanotic heart disease, 5–10 min; acyanotic heart disease, 1.3–3 hr.
Peak Effect: Cyanotic heart disease, 30 min; acyanotic heart disease, 1.5–3 hr.
Duration of Action: 1–2 hr (after infusion).
Interaction/Toxicity: Inhibits platelet aggregation; apnea at high doses.

Guidelines/Precautions

1. Use with caution in neonates with bleeding tendencies.
2. Do not use in respiratory distress syndrome.
3. Measure efficacy by monitoring blood oxygenation, arterial pressure, and blood pH.
4. Apnea occurs in 10%–12% of neonates weighing <2 kg at birth.

Principal Adverse Reactions

Cardiovascular: Hypotension, bradycardia, arrhythmias, CHF.
Pulmonary: Apnea, bronchial wheezing, respiratory depression.
CNS: Seizures, cerebral bleeding, lethargy, hypothermia.
GI: Diarrhea, gastric regurgitation, hyperbilirubinemia.
Hematologic: Disseminated intravascular coagulation, anemia, thrombocytopenia.
Renal: Anuria, hematuria.
Skeletal: Cortical proliferation of the long bones.
Other: Hyperkalemia, hypokalemia, hypoglycemia, peritonitis.

PROTAMINE SULFATE (PROTAMINE SULFATE)

Use(s): Heparin antagonist.
Dosing: Slow IV, 1 mg neutralizes 90 USP units heparin (lung) or 115 USP units heparin (intestinal mucosa); do not exceed 50 mg in any 10-min period; dose determined by dose of heparin given, route of administration, and time elapsed since it was given. Give one half of dose if 30–60 min have elapsed since IV injection of heparin and one fourth of dose if ≥2 hr have elapsed.
Elimination: Hepatic.
How Supplied: Injection: 10 mg/mL.

Pharmacology

This low molecular weight protein is rich in arginine and strongly basic. It neutralizes heparin by combining with it to form a stable complex that is devoid of anticoagulant activity. Despite the formation of this complex, the effect of heparin may persist and be responsible for continued bleeding, especially after cardiopulmonary bypass. In the absence of heparin, protamine has a weak anticoagulant effect. Rapid IV injection is associated with histamine release, peripheral vasodilation, decrease in blood pressure, and an increase in pulmonary vascular resistance.

Pharmacokinetics

Onset of Action: 30 sec–1 min.
Peak Effect: <5 min.
Duration of Action: 2 hr (dependent on body temperature).
Interaction/Toxicity: Potentiates vasodilators; severe hypotension and anaphylactoid reactions with rapid IV administration; chemically incompatible with solutions of cephalosporins and penicillin.

Guidelines/Precautions

1. Hyperheparinemia or bleeding may occur 30 min–18 hr after complete neutralization of heparin.
2. Unwise to give >100 mg over a short time unless there is certain knowledge of a larger requirement.
3. Rapid administration of protamine may result in severe hypotension and anaphylaxis.
4. Increased risk of allergic reactions in patients who are allergic to fish or who have been previously treated with protamine-containing insulin preparations and in the presence of antiprotamine antibodies in the serum of infertile or vasectomized men.
5. Patients known to be allergic to protamine and requiring heparin anticoagulation may be pretreated with histamine receptor antagonists, followed by a slow-trial IV infusion of protamine; may be allowed to recover from the heparin effect, requiring multiple blood transfusions, or may be given hexadimethrine, an alternate heparin antagonist (not available for general use in the United States).
6. Protamine may be inactivated by blood. When it is used to neutralize large doses of heparin, a heparin "rebound" may occur. More protamine should be administered in this instance.

Principal Adverse Reactions

Cardiovascular: Hypotension, hypertension, bradycardia.
Pulmonary: Pulmonary hypertension, dyspnea, bronchospasm.
Allergic: Anaphylactoid reactions, anaphylaxis, flushing.
GI: Nausea, vomiting, thrombocytopenia.

PYRIDOSTIGMINE BROMIDE (MESTINON, REGONOL)

Use(s): Reversal of nondepolarizing muscle relaxants, treatment of myasthenia gravis.
Dosing: Reversal: IV, 10–30 mg (0.1–0.25 mg/kg), preceded by atropine or glycopyrrolate (atropine IV, 0.015 mg/kg, or glycopyrrolate IV, 0.01 mg/kg).

Myasthenia gravis: PO, 60–1500 mg/day (average 600 mg/day); space doses to provide maximum relief (children, 7 mg/kg/day divided in 5–6 doses); PO-SR, 180–540 mg once daily or bid. To supplement oral dosage preoperatively and postoperatively, during labor and postpartum, during myasthenic crisis, or when oral therapy is impractical, give ⅓₀ the oral dose IM or very slow IV.

Neonates of myasthenic mothers: 0.05–0.15 mg/kg IM. Differentiate between cholinergic and myasthenic crisis in the neonates. Administration of pyridostigmine 1 hr before completion of the second stage of labor enables patients to have adequate strength during labor and provides protection to infants in the immediate postnatal state.

Elimination: Hepatic, renal.
How Supplied: Injection, 5 mg/mL; tablets: 60 mg; tablets (SR), 180 mg; oral solution, 60 mg/5 mL.

Pharmacology

This pyridine analogue of neostigmine is an anticholinesterase agent and blocks the enzyme responsible for the hydrolysis of acetylcholine. Acetylcholine levels build, thereby facilitating the transmission of impulses across the myoneural junction. In myasthenia gravis there is an increased response of skeletal muscle to repetitive impulses because of increased availability of acetylcholine. This drug has a slower onset and longer duration of action than neostimine. When used for reversal of neuromuscular blockade, the muscarinic cholinergic effects (bradycardia, salivation, GI stimulation) are prevented by the concurrent use of atropine or glycopyrrolate.

Pharmacokinetics

Onset of Action: Reversal IV: 2–5 min. Myaesthenia: IM, <15 min; PO, 20–30 min.
Peak Effect: Reversal IV: within 15 min. Myaesthenia: IM, 15 min.
Duration of Action: Reversal IV: 90 min. Myaesthenia: PO, 3–6 hr; IM, 2–4 hr.
Interaction/Toxicity: Does not antagonize and may prolong the phase 1 block of succinylcholine; antagonizes the effects of nondepolarizing muscle relaxants, such as tubocurarine, atracurium, vecuronium, pancuronium; antagonism of neuromuscular blockade is reduced by aminoglycoside antibiotics, hypothermia, hypokalemia, respiratory and metabolic acidosis; may produce bradycardia, salivation, fasciculations, GI stimulation.

Guidelines/Precautions

1. Contraindicated in patients with peritonitis or mechanical obstruction of the intestines or urinary tract.
2. Pyridostigmine overdosage may induce a cholinergic crisis characterized by nausea, vomiting, bradycardia or tachycardia, excessive salivation and sweating, bronchospasm, weakness, and paralysis.
3. Treatment of a cholinergic crisis includes discontinuation of pyridostigmine and administration of atropine (10 μg/kg IV q3–10min until muscarinic symptoms disappear) and, if necessary, pralidoxime (15 mg/kg IV over 2 min) for reversal of nicotinic symptoms. Give other supportive treatment as indicated (artificial respiration, tracheostomy, oxygen, etc.).
4. Use with caution in patients with bradycardia, bronchial asthma, cardiac arrhythmias, or peptic ulcer.

Principal Adverse Reactions

Cardiovascular: Bradycardia, AV block, nodal rhythm, hypotension.

Pulmonary: Increased bronchial secretions, bronchospasm, respiratory depression.

GI: Nausea, vomiting, diarrhea, abdominal cramps, increased peristalsis, increased salivation.

Musculoskeletal: Muscle cramps, fasciculations, weakness.

Other: Miosis, diaphoresis.

RANITIDINE (ZANTAC)

Use(s): Treatment of duodenal ulcer, gastroesophageal reflux, pathologic hypersecretory conditions; prophylaxis against acid pulmonary aspiration.

Dosing: PO, 150 mg bid; alternately, 150–300 mg at bedtime.
IV/IM, 50 mg q6–8h (dilute IV dose in 20 ml NS solution and give over 5–15 min).

Elimination: Hepatic.

How Supplied: Tablet, 150 mg, 300 mg; injection, 25 mg/mL.

Pharmacology

This histamine H_2 receptor antagonist blocks histamine-, pentagastrin-, and acetylcholine-induced secretion of hydrogen ions by gastric parietal cells. Nocturnal and food-induced gastric secretion are also inhibited. It has no significant effect on gastric emptying time, volume, or pancreatic secretions. Single oral dose of 150 mg will provide acid inhibition for 8–12 hr. Ranitidine also suppresses histamine-induced peripheral vasodilation and inotropic effects. Minimal entrance into the CNS and thus in contrast with cimetidine produces fewer side effects such as CNS dysfunction in elderly patients. Also reported to produce less inhibition of microsomal drug metabolizing enzymes and less antiandrogen effects than cimetidine.

Pharmacokinetics

Onset of Action: IV, <15 min; PO, <30 min.

Peak Effect: PO, 2–3 hr.

Duration of Action: IV, 6–8 hr; PO, 8–12 hr.
Interaction/Toxicity: Absorption decreased by concurrent antacids; may decrease absorption of diazepam; may increase hypoglycemic effect of glipizide; may interfere with warfarin clearance; bradycardia after infusion.

Guidelines/Precautions

1. Use with caution in elderly patients.
2. Full daily dose may be given at one time.

Principal Adverse Reactions

Cardiovascular: Tachycardia, bradycardia, premature ventricular beats with rapid IV injection.
Pulmonary: Bronchospasm.
CNS: Headache, depression, dizziness, confusion.
GI/Hepatic: Nausea, vomiting, hepatitis, diarrhea.
Hematologic: Leukopenia, granulocytopenia, thrombocytopenia.
Dermatologic: Erythema multiforme, alopecia.

RITODRINE HCL (YUTOPAR)

Use(s): Uterine relaxation; threatened or spontaneous abortion.
Dosing: Infusion: 0.05–0.3 mg/min (Titrate upward by 0.05 mg/min q10 min until desired response); continue infusion for at least 12 hr after cessation of uterine contractions.
PO: 10 mg q2h for 24 hr, then 10–20 mg q4–6 h (maximum dose, 120 mg/day).
Elimination: Hepatic.
How Supplied: Injection, 10 mg/mL, 15 mg/mL; tablets, 10 mg.
Dilution for Infusion: 150 mg in 500 mL NS solution (0.3 mg/mL).

Pharmacology

This β_2-adrenergic receptor agonist increases the levels of cyclic AMP in uterine smooth muscle. Calcium cellular balance is altered resulting in relaxation. β_1-Effects manifest as tachycardia, hypertension, and fluid overload because of increased sodium and water retention. Pulmonary edema may also be secondary to excessive tachycardia. IV infusion is associated with transient elevations in the levels of blood glucose, insulin, fatty acids, and a decrease in serum potassium levels. Ritodrine readily crosses the placenta, and the concentration of insulin in cord blood may be increased, resulting in neonatal hypoglycemia.

Pharmacokinetics

Onset of Action: IV, immediate.
Peak Effect: IV, <50 min; PO, 30–60 min.
Duration of Action: 1.7–2.6 hr (half-life).
Interaction/Toxicity: Increased incidence of pulmonary edema with concomitant administration of corticosteroids; potentiates cardiovascular depression of volatile anesthetics, magnesium, narcotics, diazoxide; additive effects (hypertension) with sympathomimetics and in the presence of parasympatholytics such as atropine; hypokalemia associated with infusion and also use of potassium-depleting diuretics; may increase insulin requirements in insulin-dependent diabetics; action antagonized by β-adrenergic-blocking drugs.

Guidelines/Precautions

1. Monitor glucose and electrolyte levels during infusions.
2. Contraindicated before the 20th week of pregnancy and in those conditions in which continuation of the pregnancy is hazardous to the mother or fetus, specifically, antepartum hemorrhage that demands immediate delivery, eclampsia, severe preeclampsia, intrauterine fetal death, chorioamnionitis, maternal cardiac disease, pulmonary hypertension, maternal hyperthyroidism, uncontrolled maternal diabetes mellitus, pre-existing maternal medical conditions such as pheochromocytoma, hypovolemia, bronchial asthma already treated by beta-mimetics and/or corticosteroids.
3. Frequent monitoring of maternal uterine contractions, heart rate, blood pressure, and fetal heart rate is required.
4. Monitor fluid intake. To avoid pulmonary edema, limit fluid intake to 1.5–2 L/24 hr.
5. Pulmonary edema is especially common in patients taking corticosteroids.

Principal Adverse Reactions

Cardiovascular: Tachycardia, palpitations, arrhythmias, hypertension, angina, bradycardia after drug withdrawal.
Pulmonary: Dyspnea, hyperventilation, pulmonary edema.
CNS: Tremors, headache, anxiety.
GI: Nausea, vomiting, diarrhea.
Metabolic: Hypokalemia, hyperglycemia, hyperinsulinemia.
Neonatal: Tachycardia, hypoglycemia, ileus.

SCOPOLAMINE HYDROBROMIDE
(SCOPOLAMINE HYDROBROMIDE)

Use(s): Premedication, sedation, amnesia, vagolysis, treatment of motion sickness.
Dosing: PO: 0.4–0.8 mg.
IV/IM/SC: 0.2–0.65 mg (children, 0.006 mg/kg; maximum dose, 0.3 mg); dilute with sterile water for IV administration.
Transdermal patch: 1.5 mg. Apply to postauricular skin.
Elimination: Hepatic, renal.
How Supplied: Capsules, 0.25 mg; injection, 0.3 mg/mL, 0.4 mg/mL, 0.86 mg/mL, 1 mg/mL; transdermal patch, 1.5 mg. Delivers 5 µg/hr for 72 hr; ophthalmic solution: 0.25%.

Pharmacology

This ester of the organic base scopine antagonizes the action of acetylcholine at cholinergic postganglionic nerve endings. Scopolamine has greater antisialogogue and ocular effects than atropine and lesser effects on the heart (tachycardia), bronchial smooth muscle (bronchodilation), and GI tract. The decrease in heart rate by small doses reflects a weak peripheral muscarinic cholinergic effect. It is a tertiary amine and may readily cross the blood-brain barrier, exerting effects on the CNS. Scopolamine produces a more marked and longer-lasting sedative effect than atropine, and therapeutic doses may cause drowsiness, euphoria, amnesia, and fatigue. It prevents motion sickness by inhibition of vestibular in-

put to the CNS and a direct action on the vomiting center within
the reticular formation of the brain stem.

Pharmacokinetics

Onset of Action: IV, almost immediate; IM/PO/transdermal,
Within 30 min.
Peak Effect: IV, 50–80 min; IM/PO, 2 hr; transdermal, 3 hr.
Duration of Action: IV, 2 hr; IM/PO, 4–6 hr; transdermal, 3
days.
Interaction/Toxicity: Central anticholinergic syndrome (hallucinations, delirium, coma); potentiates sedative effects of narcotics,
benzodiazepines, anticholinergics, antihistamines, volatile anesthetics.

Guidelines/Precautions

1. Treat central anticholinergic syndrome with IV physostigmine, 15–60 μg/kg.
2. Use with great caution in patients with glaucoma, coronary
   artery disease, urinary bladder neck, pyloric or intestinal obstruction.
3. May cause confusion and restlessness, particularly in the elderly and young.

Principal Adverse Reactions

Cardiovascular: Tachycardia, bradycardia (with small doses).
Pulmonary: Tachypnea.
CNS: Drowsiness, confusion, disorientation, restlessness.
GI: Constipation, paralytic ileus, nausea, vomiting, dry mouth.
Eye: Blurred vision, impairment of accommodation.
Allergic: Urticaria, anaphylaxis.

SECOBARBITAL (SECONAL)

Use(s): Premedication, sedation, hypnosis; anticonvulsant.
Dosing: Premedication and sedation: IM, 4–5 mg/kg (inject
        deep and not >250 mg in any one site); PO,
        100–300 mg (children, 2–6 mg/kg; maximum
        dose, 100 mg); rectal, 4–5 mg/kg (dilute injectable

solution with water to a concentration of 10–15 mg/
mL).

Hypnosis: IV, titrate (average dose, 50–100 mg), do
not exceed 50 mg/15 min; total dosage in excess of
250 mg is not recommended.

Anticonvulsive: 5.5 mg/kg IM or slow IV; repeat
q3–4h prn.

Elimination: Hepatic.

How Supplied: Injection, 50 mg/mL; tablets, 100 mg; capsules,
50 mg, 100 mg; rectal injection, 50 mg/mL.

Pharmacology

This short-acting barbiturate depresses the sensory cortex, decreases motor activity, alters cerebellar function, and produces
dose-dependent drowsiness, sedation, and hypnosis. It may induce paradoxical excitement in elderly persons and children and
in the presence of acute or chronic pain. Induction doses produce
respiratory depression, decreases in peripheral vascular resistance,
arterial pressure, cardiac output, and a fall in coronary perfusion
pressure.

Pharmacokinetics

Onset of Action: IV, almost immediate; PO, 10–30 min; IM/rec-
tal, 15–30 min.

Peak Effect: IV, 1 min.

Duration of Action: IV: Awakening, 15 min; sedative effect,
3–4 hr.

PO/IM/rectal: Sedative effect, 6–8 hr.

Interaction/Toxicity: Potentiates CNS and circulatory depressant
effects of narcotics, sedative hypnotics, alcohol, volatile anesthetics; decreases effects of oral anticoagulants, digoxin, β-blockers,
corticosteroids, quinidine, theophylline; actions prolonged by
MAO inhibitors, chloramphenicol; arterial or extravascular injection produces necrosis, gangrene.

Guidelines/Precautions

1. Contraindicated in patients with history of manifest or latent
   porphyria, status asthmaticus, and in the presence of acute or
   chronic pain.

2. Use with caution in patients with hypertension, hypovolemia, ischemic heart disease, acute adrenocortical insufficiency, uremia, septicemia, and for obstetric delivery.
3. Reduce doses in elderly, hypovolemic, or high-risk surgical patients and with concomitant use of narcotics and other sedatives.
4. Treat intra-arterial injection by local infiltration of phentolamine (5–10 mg in 10 mL NS solution) and, if necessary, sympathetic block.
5. Use IV route only in emergency.

Principal Adverse Reactions

Cardiovascular: Bradycardia, hypotension.
Pulmonary: Respiratory depression, apnea, laryngospasm, bronchospasm.
CNS: Somnolence, paradoxical excitement, ataxia, confusion.
GI: Nausea, vomiting, constipation, diarrhea.
Allergic: Rash, urticaria, angioneurotic edema.
Dermatologic: Necrosis, gangrene with intra-arterial injection.

SODIUM BICARBONATE (SODIUM BICARBONATE)

Use(s): Correction of metabolic acidosis, urinary alkalinization, enhancement of rate of onset and potency of local anesthetics.
Dosing: Acidosis in cardiac arrest: IV, 1 mEq/kg (followed by 0.5 mEq/kg q10min of arrest, depending on arterial blood gas values). Due to absence of proved efficacy and many adverse effects, use sodium bicarbonate only after application of more definitive and substantiated interventions such as prompt defibrillation, chest compression, endotracheal intubation, and hyperventilation with 100% O_2 and use of drugs such as epinephrine and lidocaine (these interventions take ~ 10 min).

Acidosis: Body weight (kg) × base deficit (mEq/L) × 0.3 (0.4 in infants) = bicarbonate dose (mEq). Give one half of calculated estimate; further doses should depend on clinical response. In the presence of normal renal function, achieving a total carbon dioxide content of about 20 mEq/L will be associated with a normal blood pH; (neonates and children [<2 yr], slow IV administration of a 4.2% solution of the calculated dose; maximum dose, 8 mEq/kg/day).

Bicarbonation of local anesthetics: Add 0.1 mL 8.4% sodium bicarbonate with 20 mL 0.25% bupivacaine; add 1 mL 8.4% sodium bicarbonate with 30 mL 2%–3% chloroprocaine; add 1 mL 8.4% sodium bicarbonate with 10 mL 0.5%–2% lidocaine; add 1 mL 8.4% sodium bicarbonate with 10 mL 1%–3% mepivacaine; add 1 mL 8.4% sodium bicarbonate with 10 mL 0.5%–2% prilocaine; Do not use if the local anesthetic precipitates out of the solution.

Alkalinization of urine: 48 mEq (4 g) initially, then 12–24 mEq (1–2 g) q4h; dosage of 30–48 mEq (2.5–4 g) q4h may be required in some patients.

Elimination: Renal.

How Supplied: Injection: Adult, 8.4% (1 mEq/mL); pediatric, 7.5% (0.892 mEq/mL), 5% (0.6 mEq/mL); children <2 yr and neonates, 4.2% (0.5 mEq/mL); solution sterile to adjust pH of injections 4.2% (0.5 mEq/mL) and 4% (0.48 mEq/mL).

Tablets: 300 mg, 325 mg, 600 mg, 650 mg.

Pharmacology

Dissociates in water to provide sodium and bicarbonate ions. Buffers excess hydrogen ion concentration and raises blood pH. One gram provides 11.9 mEq sodium and 11.9 mEq bicarbonate. Urinary alkalinization is useful in the treatment of certain drug intoxications (i.e., barbiturates, salicylates, lithium, methyl alcohol), in hemolytic reactions to diminish nephrotoxicity of blood pigments, and in methotrexate therapy to prevent nephrotoxicity. Bicarbonation of local anesthetics increases the pH and enhances rate of onset and potency. A big increase in pH may precipitate the local anesthetic out of solution as drug base.

Pharmacokinetics

Onset of Action: 2–10 min.
Peak Effect: 10–30 min.
Duration of Action: 30–60 min.
Interaction/Toxicity: Increases risks of solute overload with coadministration of parenteral fluids, especially those containing sodium, in patients receiving corticosteroids or corticotropin; chemical incompatibility with solutions containing calcium; increases end-tidal CO_2; urinary alkalinization increases half-lives and duration of action of quinidine, amphetamines, ephedrine, and pseudoephedrine; increased renal clearance of tetracyclines,

especially doxycycline; extravasation may cause tissue necrosis, sloughing; metabolic acidosis may occur with excessive, too rapid administration and in patients with hypokalemia or hypochloremia; carpopedal spasms as pH rises in patients with coexistent hypocalcemia; hypokalemia from intracellular shift of potassium may occur with excessive administration and predispose to cardiac arrhythmias.

Guidelines/Precautions

1. Avoid overdosage and alkalosis by giving repeated small doses and monitoring pH.
2. Use cautiously in patients with CHF or other edematous or sodium-retaining states, as well as in patients with oliguria or anuria.
3. Treat electrolyte imbalances before or concomitantly with bicarbonate.
4. In neonates and children (<2 yr), rapid injection of hypertonic sodium bicarbonate solutions may produce hypernatremia, decrease in cerebrospinal fluid, and possibly intracranial hemorrhage.
5. Treat extravasation by prompt elevation of the part, warmth, and local injection of lidocaine or hyaluronidase.
6. Control symptoms of alkalosis (tetany, hyperirritability) by parenteral injection of calcium gluconate or, if severe, IV infusion of 2.14% ammonium chloride solution. Sodium chloride (0.9%) IV or potassium chloride may be indicated if there is hypokalemia.
7. Liberation of CO_2 and its rapid intracellular diffusion after sodium bicarbonate administration worsen intracellular acidosis during cardiopulmonary resuscitation. Increased arterial PCO_2 (and the paradoxical acidosis) is a rapidly acting and potent negative inotrope. On the contrary, the negative inotropic effect of metabolic acidosis is slower in onset and may not be fully manifest until 30 min have elapsed from onset of acidosis to a magnitude equivalent to that induced more rapidly by CO_2.

Principal Adverse Reactions

Cardiovascular: Peripheral edema, arrhythmias.
Pulmonary: Pulmonary edema.

CNS: Intracranial hemorrhage.
Metabolic: Alkalosis, hypernatremia, hypokalemia, hyperosmolality, intracellular/CSF/central venous acidosis, inhibition of oxygen release to the tissues.
Dermatologic: Necrosis, sloughing with extravasation.

SODIUM CITRATE (SHOHL'S SOLUTION, BICITRA)

Use(s): Antacid, premedication (aspiration prophylaxis), systemic alkalinization.
Dosing: PO: 15–30 mL diluted with 15–30 mL water as single dose. Each mL contains 1 mEq sodium and is equivalent to 1 mEq bicarbonate.
Elimination: Hepatic.
How Supplied: Unit dose: 15 mL, 30 mL, 120 mL, 1 pint, 1 gallon.

Pharmacology

Nonparticulate acid-neutralizing buffer. Fast acting and useful in raising the pH value of gastric acid. 15 mL will neutralize and buffer 117 mL of 0.1N HCl to pH 2.5.

Pharmacokinetics

Onset of Action: Almost immediate.
Peak Effect: Few minutes.
Duration of Action: 2 hr.
Interaction/Toxicity: May induce alkalosis, especially in the presence of hypocalcemia.

Guidelines/Precautions

1. Contraindicated in patients on sodium-restricted diet or with severe renal impairment.
2. Because of high sodium content (1 mEq/mL), use cautiously in patients with cardiac failure, hypertension, impaired renal function, peripheral and pulmonary edema, and toxemia of pregnancy.

Principal Adverse Reactions

Cardiovascular: Seizures.
GI: Nausea, vomiting, diarrhea.
Metabolic: Alkalosis.

SODIUM NITROPRUSSIDE (NIPRIDE, NITROPRESS)

Use(s): Antihypertensive, controlled hypotension, treatment of cardiogenic pulmonary edema, pre–cardiac transplant evaluation.
Dosing: Infusion: 10–300 µg/min (0.25–10 µg/kg/min). Maximum dose, 10 µg/kg/min for 10 min or chronic infusion of 0.5 µg/kg/min. Wrap infusion bag in aluminium foil or opaque material to protect from light.
Elimination: Hepatic.
How Supplied: 5 mL vial containing 50 mg.
Dilution for Infusion: 50 mg in 2–3 mL D_5W, then in 250 mL D_5W (200 µg/mL).

Pharmacology

Nitroprusside is a potent peripheral vasodilator that acts on both arterial and venous smooth muscle. Its vasodilating properties may result from the generation of nitric oxide, which may be endothelial-derived relaxing factor (EDRF). It lacks significant effects on other smooth muscle such as the uterus or duodenum. The decreased peripheral vascular resistance reduces blood pressure and may activate baroreceptor-mediated reflex tachycardia. It may alter pulmonary ventilation/perfusion ratio (thus increasing shunting) and increase cerebral blood flow. Nitroprusside is rapidly metabolized to cyanide, which is converted to thiocyanate by the enzyme rhodanase in the liver and kidney. This detoxification reaction depends on the availability of a sulfur donor (endogenous thiosulfate).

Pharmacokinetics

Onset of Action: 30–60 sec.
Peak Effect: 1–2 min.

Duration of Action: 1–10 min.

Interaction/Toxicity: Hypotensive effects potentiated by volatile anesthetics, ganglionic blocking agents, other antihypertensive and circulatory depressants; cyanide toxicity manifested by tachyphylaxis, elevated mixed venous Po_2, metabolic acidosis; thiocyanate toxicity (>10 mg/100 mL) manifested by skeletal muscle weakness, nausea, mental confusion, hypothyroidism.

Guidelines/Precautions

1. There is risk of cyanide toxicity even at relatively low doses, and appropriate monitoring is required. Treat cyanide toxicity by immediate discontinuation of nitroprusside. Administer B_{12} (1 g/50 mg of nitroprusside) or amyl nitrite inhalation for 15–30 sec each minute until a slow IV administration of sodium nitrite 5 mg/kg (3% solution) over 5 min to convert hemoglobin to methemoglobin. Then follow with IV sodium thiosulfate (150 mg/kg in 50 mL D_5W over 15 min).
2. Monitor plasma thiocyanate concentrations in any patient receiving therapy for >48 hr. Thiocyanate retention is more likely to occur in patients with impaired renal function or hyponatremia and may manifest with symptoms of hypothyroidism. The thiocyanate ion is readily removed by peritoneal or hemodialysis.
3. Contraindicated in patients with compensatory hypertension, such as arteriovenous shunts, coarctation of the aorta, and those with inadequate cerebral circulation.
4. Administer with a calibrated infusion pump.

Principal Adverse Reactions

Cardiovascular: Hypotension, collapse, palpitations, tachycardia.
CNS: Headache, apprehension, raised intracranial pressure.
GI: Nausea, retching.
Hematologic: Methemoglobinemia.
Other: Cyanide toxicity, hypothyroidism, antiplatelet effect, methemoglobinemia.

SUCCINYLCHOLINE CHLORIDE (ANECTINE, QUELICIN, SUCOSTRIN)

Use(s): Depolarizing muscle relaxant.
Dosing: IV, 0.7–1 mg/kg (1.5 mg/kg with nondepolarizer pretreatment); neonates and infants, 2–3 mg/kg; children 1–2 mg/kg.
      Deep IM, 2.5–4 mg/kg (maximum dose, 150 mg); infusion, 0.5–10 mg/min (titrate to desired response).
Elimination: Plasma pseudocholinesterase.
How Supplied: Injection, 20 mg/mL, 50 mg/mL, 100 mg/mL; powder for injection, 100 mg, 500 mg, 1 g/vial with diluent.
Dilution for Infusion: 250 mg in 250 mL D_5W or NS solution (1 mg/mL).

Pharmacology

Ultra-short-acting depolarizing skeletal muscle relaxant. Like acetylcholine, it combines with cholinergic receptors of the motor end plate to produce depolarization observed as fasciculations. Neuromuscular transmission is then inhibited as long as an adequate concentration of succinylcholine remains at the receptor site; the neuromuscular block produces a flaccid paralysis. It has no effect on consciousness, pain threshold, or cerebration and no direct effect on the uterus or other smooth muscles. It increases intraocular pressure. Barrier pressure is maintained, with elevation of both intragastric and lower esophageal sphincter pressure. When given over a long period, the characteristic, depolarizing neuromuscular block (phase I block) may change to a block that superficially resembles a nondepolarizing block (phase II block). This may be associated with prolonged hypoventilation. After confirmation of phase II block by peripheral nerve stimulation (train-of-four fade, post-tetanic facilitation) observe spontaneous recovery of the twitch for 20–30 min, then reverse with anticholinesterase, e.g., neostigmine, combined with an anticholinergic agent (e.g., glycopyrrolate or atropine). A phase I block will be potentiated. Histamine release occurs but is rarely of clinical significance. Initial cardiac effects reflect actions at autonomic ganglia (elevations in heart rate and blood pressure). Subsequent cardiac effects at higher doses (sinus bradycardia, junctional rhythm) reflect actions at cardiac muscarinic cholinergic receptors.

Pharmacokinetics

Onset of Action: IV, 30–60 sec; IM, 2–3 min.
Peak Effect: IV, 60 sec.
Duration of Action: IV 4–6 min; IM, 10–30 min.
Interaction/Toxicity: Prolonged blockade in patients with hypokalemia or hypocalcemia, low plasma pseudocholinesterase, myasthenia gravis, and patients receiving phenelzine, β-adrenergic blockers, procainamide, lidocaine, magnesium, oxytocin, anticholinesterases, trimethaphan, volatile anesthetics; unpredictable response in myasthenia gravis; bradycardia after second IV injection, especially in children; increased sensitivity to succinylcholine during pregnancy secondary to decreased pseudocholinesterase; incompatible with alkaline solutions and will precipitate thiopental sodium.

Guidelines/Precautions

1. Monitor response with peripheral nerve stimulator.
2. Abrupt onset of malignant hyperthermia may be triggered by succinylcholine. Early premonitory signs include muscle rigidity, especially jaw muscles, tachycardia and tachypnea unresponsive to increased depth of anesthesia, evidence of increased oxygen consumption and carbon dioxide production (change in color and increased temperature of the CO_2 absorber), rising body temperature, and metabolic acidosis.
3. Development of masseter muscle spasm after administration of succinylcholine may be associated with malignant hyperthermia susceptibility. However, it may be due to an insufficient dose of succinylcholine (especially in children). The anesthetic may be continued without triggering agents and the patient evaluated for malignant hyperthermia. The development of an increase in muscle tone, rising body temperature, and cardiac arrhythmias suggests that the patient is undergoing a hypermetabolic episode. The anesthetic needs to be abandoned and treatment begun for malignant hyperthermia.
4. Use with caution in patients with fractures, muscle spasm caused by additional trauma from fasciculations, or cardiovascular, hepatic, pulmonary, metabolic, or renal disorders.

5. Repeated administration at short intervals (<5 min) are associated with bradycardia. Bradycardia may be prevented by atropine, thiopental, ganglionic blocking drugs, and nondepolarizing muscle relaxants.

6. Elevates serum potassium (0.3–0.5 mEq/L in normal patients). Alarming levels of potassium (as high as 11 mEq/L) along with cardiovascular collapse may occur when succinycholine is used in patients with severe burns, hyperkalemia, electrolyte imbalance, severe trauma, paraplegia, spinal cord injury, degenerative or dystrophic neuromuscular disease.

7. Increases both intragastric and gastroesophageal sphincter pressure. Fasciculations may increase potential for regurgitation and possible aspiration.

8. Administration of succinylcholine soon after an anticholinesterase, e.g., neostigmine or pyridostigmine, will produce a prolonged neuromuscular blockade (up to 60 min). This is partly due to inhibition of plasma pseudocholinesterase and delayed metabolism of succinylcholine.

9. Prolonged respiratory paralysis in patients with low plasma pseudocholinesterase, as in severe liver disease or cirrhosis, burns, cancer, pregnancy, dehydration, collagen disease, and abnormal body temperatures, in patients receiving pancuronium, MAO inhibitors, neostigmine, oral contraceptives, chlorpromazine, or in those with a recessive hereditary trait. Administer minimal doses (test dose, 5–10 mg) with extreme care.

10. Contraindicated in patients with genetic disorders of plasma pseudocholinesterases, familial history of malignant hyperthermia, myopathies associated with elevated creatine phosphokinase (CPK) values; acute narrow-angle glaucoma, penetrating eye injuries, hypersensitivity to succinylcholine.

Principal Adverse Reactions

Cardiovascular: Hypotension, bradycardia, arrhythmias, tachycardia, hypertension.
Pulmonary: Hypoventilation, apnea, bronchospasm.
GI: Excess salivation, increased intragastric and lower esophageal sphincter tone.
Allergic: Anaphylactic reactions, rash.

Musculoskeletal: Prolonged block, inadequate block, muscle soreness.
Other: Hyperkalemia, malignant hyperthermia, myoglobinemia, increased intraocular pressure.

SUFENTANIL CITRATE (SUFENTA)*

Use(s): Analgesia, anesthesia.
Dosing: Analgesia: IV/IM, 0.2–0.6 µg/kg; intranasal, 1.5–3 µg/kg (use undiluted injectate solution for intranasal route).
   Induction: IV, 2–10 µg/kg.
   Infusion: 0.01–0.05 µg/kg/min.
   Epidural: Bolus, 0.2–0.6 µg/kg; infusion, 5–30 µg/hr (0.2–0.6 µg/kg/hr).
   Spinal: 0.02–0.08 µg/kg.
   Patient-controlled analgesia: IV (bolus), 2–10 µg; (infusion), 2–5 µg/hr; (lockout interval), 3–10 min; Epidural (bolus), 4 µg; (infusion), 6 µg/hr; (Lockout interval), 10–20 min.
Elimination: Hepatic.
How Supplied: Injection: 50 µg/mL.
Dilution for Infusion: IV, 500 µg in 100 mL NS (5 µg/mL); epidural, 100 µg in 100 mL local anesthetic or (preservative-free) NS solution (1 µg/mL).

Pharmacology

This drug is a thiamyl analogue of fentanyl with 5–7 times the analgesic potency. Sufentanil attenuates the hemodynamic response to endotracheal intubation and surgical manipulation (e.g., incision). Cardiovascular effects are generally similar to those of fentanyl. It may produce bradycardia sufficient to decrease cardiac output, and depression of ventilation may follow administration. It causes a decrease in cerebral metabolic requirements for oxygen. Has no clinically significant effect on cerebral blood flow or ICP.

---

*For epidural/intrathecal precautions, see Alfentanil, Guidelines/Precautions, items 5 and 6, pp 4–5.

Pharmacokinetics

Onset of Action: IV, immediate; intranasal, <5 min; epidural and spinal, 4–10 min.
Peak Effect: IV, 3–5 min; intranasal, 10 min; epidural and spinal, <30 min.
Duration of Action: IV, 20–45 min; IM, 2–4 hr; epidural and spinal, 4–8 hr.
Interaction/Toxicity: Circulatory- and ventilatory-depressant effects potentiated by other narcotics, sedatives, nitrous oxide, volatile anesthetics; ventilatory-depressant effects potentiated by MAO inhibitors, phenothiazines, and tricyclic antidepressants; analgesia enhanced by α_2-agonists (e.g., clonidine, epinephrine), skeletal muscle rigidity in higher dosages sufficient to interfere with ventilation; increased incidences of bradycardia with use of vecuronium.

Guidelines/Precautions

1. In hemodynamically stable patients, analgesic doses may be given 2–4 min prior to laryngoscopy to attenuate the pressor response to intubation. Requirements for induction agents, e.g., thiopental sodium, may be decreased.
2. Reduce doses in elderly, hypovolemic, high-risk patients, and with concomitant use of sedatives and other narcotics. Incremental doses should be determined from effect of initial dose.
3. Narcotic effect reversed with naloxone ($\geq$0.2–0.4 mg IV). Duration of reversal may be shorter than duration of narcotic effect.
4. May produce a dose-related rigidity of skeletal muscles.
5. Crosses the placental barrier; usage in labor may produce depression of respiration in the neonate. Resuscitation may be required; have naloxone available.

Principal Adverse Reactions

Cardiovascular: Hypotension, bradycardia.
Pulmonary: Respiratory depression, apnea.
CNS: Dizziness, sedation, euphoria, dysphoria, anxiety.
GI: Nausea, vomiting, delayed gastric emptying, biliary tract spasm.
Musculoskeletal: Muscle rigidity.

TERBUTALINE SULFATE (BRETHAIRE, BRICANYL)

Use(s): Bronchodilator, inhibition of premature labor.
Dosing: Bronchodilator: SC, 0.25 mg (may repeat in 15–30 min; do not exceed 0.5 mg in 4 hr) inhalation, 2 breaths separated by 60 sec q4–6h; PO, 2.5–5 mg tid.

Inhibition of premature labor (unlabeled use): Infusion IV, 10–80 μg/min (titrate upward), maintain minimum effective doses for 4 hr; PO, 2.5 mg q4–6h.
Elimination: Hepatic.
How Supplied: Injection, 1 mg/mL; aerosol, Each actuation delivers 0.2 mg; tablets, 2.5 mg, 5 mg.

Pharmacology

This β_2-adrenergic receptor agonist relieves acute bronchospasm in acute and chronic obstructive pulmonary disease. β_1-effects are manifest as tachycardia and hypertension. Continuous IV infusion as used to stop uterine contractions in premature labor has been associated with maternal tachycardia, pulmonary edema, hypoglycemia, hypokalemia, and neonatal hypoglycemia.

Pharmacokinetics

Onset of Action: SC: 5–15 min; PO, <30 min; inhalation, 5–30 min.
Peak Effect: SC, 30–60 min; PO, 2–3 hr; inhalation, 1–2 hr.
Duration of Action: SC, 90 min–4 hr; PO, 4–8 hr; inhalation, 3–6 hr.
Interaction/Toxicity: Effects antagonized by β-blockers; increased risk of arrhythmias in patients receiving volatile anesthetics, increased risk of hypokalemia in patients receiving potassium-depleting diuretics; pulmonary edema associated with continuous infusion.

Guidelines/Precautions

1. Unlabeled use for management of preterm labor.
2. Use with caution in patients with hypertension, ischemic heart

disease, arrhythmias, diabetes mellitus, hyperthyroidism, seizures, and those susceptible to hypokalemia.
3. Paradoxical bronchoconstriction has occasionally occurred with repeated excessive use of inhalation preparations.
4. Excessive use may lead to β-agonist cardiomyopathy.
5. Contraindicated in patients with hypersensitivity to terbutaline or other sympathomimetic amines.

Principal Adverse Reactions

Cardiovascular: Tachycardia, palpitations, hypertension, arrhythmias.
Pulmonary: Dyspnea, pulmonary edema.
CNS: Tremors, dizziness, headache.
GI: Nausea, vomiting, diarrhea.
Metabolic: Hypokalemia, hyperglycemia, hypoglycemia, hyperinsulinemia.

TETRACAINE (PONTOCAINE)*

Use(s): Regional and topical anesthesia.
Dosing: Spinal: Bolus/infusion, 5–20 mg (children, 0.4 mg/kg, with a minimum of 1 mg); add 10–20 μg epinephrine if desired (1% solution); dilute dose with equal volume of supplied dextrose solution (hyperbaric), cerebrospinal fluid (isobaric), or sterile water (hypobaric). Solutions containing preservatives should not be used for spinal block.
　　　Spray, topical (2% solution): Apply for 1 sec (never >2 sec); average expulsion rate of residue from spray, 200 mg/sec.
　　　Maximum safe dose: 1–1.5 mg/kg without epinephrine; 2.5 mg/kg with epinephrine.
Elimination: Plasma cholinesterase.
How Supplied: Injection: 1% with 10% dextrose, 0.2% in 6% dextrose, 0.3% in 6% dextrose; powder for reconstitution: 20 mg.

*For additional precautions, see Bupivacaine, Guidelines/Precautions, items 8 to 10, p 20.

Pharmacology

This ester of PABA is a potent long-acting local anesthetic. It stabilizes the neuronal membrane and prevents initiation and transmission of nerve impulses. It has a prolonged duration of action compared with procaine and chloroprocaine secondary to a much slower rate of hydrolysis by plasma cholinesterase. The duration of action may be further prolonged by the addition of vasoconstrictor drugs to delay systemic absorption. High plasma levels may produce seizures and cardiovascular collapse secondary to a decrease in peripheral vascular resistance and direct myocardial depression.

Pharmacokinetics

Onset of Action: Infiltration, 15 min; spinal, <10 min.
Peak Effect: Infiltration and spinal: 15 min–1 hr.
Duration of Action: Infiltration, 2–3 hr; spinal, 1.25–3.0 hr.
Interaction/Toxicity: Prolongs the effect of succinylcholine; metabolite (PABA) inhibits the action of sulfonamides; toxicity enhanced by cimetidine, anticholinesterases (which inhibit degradation); plasma levels >8mcg/mL associated with seizures, respiratory and cardiac depression; duration of regional anesthesia prolonged by vasoconstrictor agents, e.g., epinephrine.

Guidelines/Precautions

1. Not for injection.
2. Do not use on eyes.
3. To minimize systemic absorption, do not apply topically to large areas of denuded or inflamed tissue.
4. Use with caution in patients with severe disturbances of cardiac rhythm, shock, or heart block.
5. Reduce doses for spinal anesthesia in obstetric, elderly, hypovolemic, and high-risk patients and those with increased intra-abdominal pressure.
6. Cauda equina syndrome with permanent neurologic deficit has occurred in patients receiving >20 mg 1% tetracaine solution with a continuous spinal technique.
7. Potential for allergic reaction with repeated use.
8. Contraindicated in patients with hypersensitivity to tetracaine or ester-type local anesthetics.

Principal Adverse Reactions

Cardiovascular: Hypotension, bradycardia, heart block, arrhythmias, peripheral vasodilation.
Pulmonary: Respiratory impairment or paralysis.
CNS: Postspinal headache, tinnitus, seizures, blurred vision, restlessness.
Allergic: Urticaria, erythema, angioneurotic edema
Spinal: High spinal, loss of perineal sensation and sexual function, backache, weakness and paralysis of the lower extremities, loss of sphincter control, slowing of labor, cranial nerve palsies, meningitis.

THIOPENTAL SODIUM (PENTOTHAL)

Use(s): Induction agent, supplementation of regional anesthesia, anticonvulsant, reduction of elevated intracranial pressure.
Dosing: IV, 3–5 mg/kg (children, 5–6 mg/kg; infants, 7–8 mg/kg); rectal, 25 mg/kg.
Elimination: Hepatic.
How Supplied: Injection, 250 mg, 400 mg, 500 mg syringes; vials with diluent 500 mg, 1 g; kits with 1, 2.5, 5 g; rectal suspension, 400 mg/g suspension.

Pharmacology

This ultra-short-acting thiobarbiturate depresses the CNS and induces hypnosis and anesthesia but not analgesia. Recovery after a short dose is rapid, with some somnolence and anterograde amnesia. Because of the high lipid solubility and slow elimination, repeated IV doses lead to a cumulative drug effect. The drug produces respiratory depression and hemodynamic effects, including a decrease in systemic vascular resistance, arterial pressure, cardiac output, and a fall in coronary perfusion pressure. Histamine release can occur, and allergic reactions most likely represent anaphylaxis.

Pharmacokinetics

Onset of Action: IV, 10–20 sec.
Peak Effect: IV, 30 sec.

Duration of Action: IV, 5–15 min (awakening).

Interaction/Toxicity: Potentiates CNS and circulatory depressant effects of narcotics, sedative hypnotics, alcohol, volatile anesthetics; decreases effects of oral anticoagulants, digoxin, β-blockers, corticosteroids, quinidine, theophylline; actions prolonged by MAO inhibitors, chloramphenicol; incompatible with solutions of succinylcholine, tubocurarine, or other drugs with an acid pH; arterial or extravascular injection (especially with concentrations >5%) produces necrosis, gangrene.

Guidelines/Precautions

1. Treat intra-arterial or extravascular injection by local infiltration of phentolamine (5–10 mg in 10 mL NS solution), injection into the artery of a dilute solution of papaverine (40–80 mg), or 10 mL 1% procaine to inhibit smooth muscle spasm. If necessary, perform sympathetic block of the brachial plexus or stellate ganglion.
2. Shivering after pentothal anesthesia is a thermal reaction caused by increased sensitivity to cold. Treatment consists of warming the patient with blankets, maintaining room temperature, and administering chlorpromazine or methylphenidate.
3. Contraindicated in patients with status asthmaticus, acute intermittent porphyria, variegate porphyria, hereditary coproporphyria.
4. Use with caution in patients with hypertension, hypovolemia, ischemic heart disease, acute adrenocortical insufficiency, uremia, septicemia.
5. Reduce doses in elderly, hypovolemic, high-risk surgical patients, and with concomitant use of narcotics and sedatives.

Principal Adverse Reactions

Cardiovascular: Circulatory depression, arrhythmias.
Pulmonary: Respiratory depression, apnea, laryngospasm, bronchospasm.
CNS: Emergence delirium, prolonged somnolence and recovery, headache.
GI: Nausea, emesis, salivation.
Dermatologic: Thrombophlebitis, necrosis, gangrene.
Allergic: Erythema, pruritus, urticaria, anaphylactic reactions.
Other: Skeletal muscle hyperactivity, shivering.

TRIMETHAPHAN CAMSYLATE (ARFONAD)

Use(s): Vasodilator, controlled hypotension, acute treatment of hypertensive emergencies.
Dosing: Infusion: 0.5–4 mg/min. Children: 10–150 μg/kg/min.
Elimination: Plasma cholinesterase.
How Supplied: Injection: 50 mg/mL.
Dilution for Infusion: 1500 mg in 500 mL D_5W (3 mg/mL). Do not use other diluents.

Pharmacology

Trimethaphan blocks nicotinic ganglionic receptors. It acts rapidly but so briefly that it must be given by continuous IV infusion. Directly relaxes capacitance vessels, blocks autonomic nervous system reflexes, and lowers blood pressure by decreasing cardiac output and reducing peripheral vascular resistance. Histamine release does not contribute to the reduction in blood pressure, and there is no association with increases in plasma concentrations of catecholamines and renin reflecting the effect of ganglionic blockade. Increases in heart rate most likely reflect parasympathetic blockade. Ganglionic blockade is caused by occupation of receptors normally responsive to acetylcholine, as well as stabilization of postsynaptic membranes against the actions of acetylcholine released from presynaptic nerve endings. Decreases cerebral blood flow and evokes smaller increases in intracranial pressure compared with nitroprusside or nitroglycerin.

Pharmacokinetics

Onset of Action: Immediate.
Peak Effect: 1–2 min.
Duration of Action: 10–30 min.
Interaction/Toxicity: Additive hypotensive effects with other antihypertensives, volatile and spinal anesthetics, sedative hypnotics, narcotics, diuretics; inhibits plasma cholinesterase and may prolong the duration of succinylcholine; potentiates nondepolarizing muscle relaxants, e.g., vecuronium.

Guidelines/Precautions

1. Contraindicated when there is inadequate availability of fluids, inability to replace blood for technical reasons, and in

conditions when hypotension may subject the patient to undue risk (e.g., hypovolemia, anemia, shock).
2. Use with caution in patients with arteriosclerosis, cardiac disease, hepatic or renal disease, degenerative disease of the CNS, Addison's disease, diabetes mellitus, or those receiving corticosteroids.
3. Mydriasis produced by trimethaphan may interfere with neurologic evaluation of the patient after neurosurgery.
4. Tachyphylaxis may occur, requiring increasing doses to maintain effect.
5. Placental transfer of drug may result in fetal toxicity.

Principal Adverse Reactions

Cardiovascular: Hypotension, tachycardia.
Pulmonary: Respiratory depression, arrest.
CNS: Decreased cerebral blood flow.
GU: Urinary retention.
GI: Ileus.
Eye: Mydriasis.
Allergic: Urticaria, pruritus, anaphylactic reaction.

VASOPRESSIN (PITRESSIN)

Use(s): Diagnosis and treatment of diabetes insipidus, treatment of GI hemorrhage, hemophilia, control of postoperative ileus.
Dosing: Diabetes insipidus: SC/IM, 5–10 units bid or tid prn.
  GI hemorrhage: Infusion, 0.2–0.4 units/min; maximum dose, 0.9 units/min.
Elimination: Renal, hepatic.
How Supplied: Injection: vasopressin, 20 units/mL; vasopressin tannate, 5 units/mL (not for IV use).
Dilution for Infusion: 200 units of vasopressin in 250 mL D_5W or NS solution (0.8 unit/mL).

Pharmacology

Vasopressin is a synthetic analogue of arginine vasopressin, the naturally occurring ADH. The antidiuretic action is ascribed to increasing the reabsorption of water by the renal tubules. Produces contraction of the smooth muscle of the GI tract and vascular bed. Enhanced GI motility may manifest as abdominal pain, nausea, and vomiting. Direct effect on vascular smooth muscle is not antagonized by denervation or adrenergic blocking drugs. Vasoconstriction and increased blood pressure occur only with doses that are much larger than those administered for the treatment of diabetes insipidus. Small doses may produce selective vasoconstriction of coronary arteries, myocardial ischemia, and in some instances, myocardial infarction. Ventricular arrhythmias may accompany these cardiac effects. Increases circulating plasma concentration of factor VIII and may be beneficial in the management of severe hemophilia particularly to reduce bleeding associated with surgery. Prolonged use may result in antibody formation and a shorter duration of action.

Pharmacokinetics

Onset of Action: IM/SC, Almost immediate (antidiuretic effect).
Peak Effect: IM/SC, 30–60 min (antidiuretic effect).
Duration of Action: IM/SC, 2–8 hr (antidiuretic effect); infusion 30–60 min (pressor response).
Interaction/Toxicity: Antidiuretic effect potentiated by carbamazepine, chlorpropamide, clofibrate, urea, fludrocortisone, tricyclic antidepressants; decreased by demeclocycline, norepinephrine, lithium, heparin, alcohol; sensitivity to pressor effect increased by ganglionic blocking agents.

Guidelines/Precautions

1. Use cautiously in the presence of epilepsy, migraine, asthma, heart failure, or any state in which a rapid addition to extracellular water may constitute a hazard.
2. Water intoxication may be treated with water restriction and temporary withdrawal of vasopressin until polyuria occurs. Severe water intoxication may require osmotic diuresis with mannitol, hypertonic dextrose, or urea alone or with furosemide.

Principal Adverse Reaction

Pulmonary: Cardiac arrest, circumoral pallor.
CNS: Tremors, vertigo, pounding in head.
GI: Abdominal cramps, nausea, vomiting.
Allergic: Anaphylaxis.
Other: Water intoxication.

VECURONIUM BROMIDE (NORCURON)

Use(s): Nondepolarizing muscle relaxant.
Dosing: IV (paralyzing), 0.08–0.1 mg/kg.
        Pretreatment/maintenance, IV, 0.01–0.02 mg/kg.
        Infusion, 1–2 μg/kg/min.
Elimination: Hepatic, renal.
How Supplied: Injection, 10 mg/5 mL, 10 mg/10 mL with diluent; use within 8 hr after reconstitution.
Dilution for Infusion: 20 mg in 100 mL D_5W (0.2 mg/mL).

Pharmacology

This monoquaternary analogue of pancuronium is a nondepolarizing neuromuscular blocking agent of intermediate duration. It competes for cholinergic receptors at the motor end plate. It is one third more potent than pancuronium, but its duration of neuromuscular activity is shorter and recovery more rapid. The time to onset and duration of maximum effect increase with increasing doses. Repeated doses have minimal cumulative effect on duration of blockade. There are no clinically significant changes in hemodynamic parameters. It does not release histamine.

Pharmacokinetics

Onset of Action: <3 min.
Peak Effect: 3–5 min.
Duration of Action: 25–30 min.
Interaction/Toxicity: Potentiated by prior administration of succinylcholine, volatile anesthetics, aminoglycoside, antibiotics, local anesthetics, loop diuretics, magnesium, lithium, ganglionic blocking drugs, hypothermia, hypokalemia, respiratory acidosis; recurrent paralysis with quinidine; enhanced neuromuscular blockade in patients with myasthenia gravis or inadequate adrenocortical function; effects antagonized by anticholinesterase inhibitors such as neostigmine, edrophonium, pyridostigmine; increased resistance or reversal of effects with use of theophylline and in patients with burn injury and paresis.

Guidelines/Precautions

1. Monitor response with peripheral nerve stimulator to minimize risk of overdosage.

2. Reverse effects with anticholinesterases such as pyridostigmine bromide, neostigmine, or edrophonium in conjunction
   with atropine or glycopyrrolate.
3. Pretreatment doses may induce a degree of neuromuscular
   blockade sufficient to cause hypoventilation in some patients.

Principal Adverse Reactions

Cardiovascular: Bradycardia.
Pulmonary: Hypoventilation, apnea.
Musculoskeletal: Inadequate block, prolonged block.

VERAPAMIL HCL (CALAN, ISOPTIN)

Use(s): Treatment of supraventricular tachyarrhythmias, angina;
antihypertensive.
Dosing: Arrhythmia: IV, 5–10 mg (0.07–0.25 mg/kg) (give
over 2 min; may repeat dose 30 min later, if necessary); PO (digitalized patients), 240–320 mg/day in divided doses tid or qid
q6–8h; (nondigitalized patients), 240–480 mg/day in divided
doses tid or qid q6–8h.

  Angina: PO, 40–120 mg tid.

  Antihypertensive: PO, 40–80 mg tid; PO-SR 120–240
mg daily. IV, 2.5–10 mg (0.05–0.2 mg/kg). Titrate to patient
response.
Elimination: Renal.
How Supplied: Injection, 2.5 mg/mL. Tablets, 40 mg, 80 mg,
120 mg (SR), 240 mg.

Pharmacology

Verapamil is a calcium channel blocker that selectively inhibits
the transmembrane influx of calcium ions into cardiac muscle and
smooth muscle. The antiarrhythmic effect is caused by inhibition
of calcium influx through the slow channel in cells of the cardiac
conduction system. It slows AV conduction and prolongs the effective refractory period within the AV node in a rate-related
manner. It reduces ventricular rate in atrial flutter or fibrillation,
interrupts reentry at the AV node, and restores normal sinus

rhythm in patients with paroxysmal supraventricular tachycardia. Verapamil increases antegrade conduction across accessory by-pass tracts, which may result in an increase in the ventricular response rate. It decreases myocardial contractility, systemic vascular resistance, and arterial pressure. Decreased myocardial demand accounts for the effectiveness in the treatment of angina pectoris. It increases intracranial pressure.

Pharmacokinetics

Onset of Action: IV, 2–5 min; PO, 30 min.
Peak Effect: IV, within 10 min; PO, 1.2–2 hr.
Duration of Action: IV, 30–60 min; PO, 3–7 hr (half-life).
Interaction/Toxicity: Potentiates effects of depolarizing and nondepolarizing muscle relaxants; additive cardiovascular depressant effects with use of volatile anesthetics, other antihypertensives such as diuretics, ACE inhibitors, vasodilators; increases toxicity of digoxin, benzodiazepines, carbamazepine, oral hypoglycemics, and possibly quinidine and theophylline; cardiac failure, AV conduction disturbances, and sinus bradycardia with concurrent use of β-blockers; severe hypotension and bradycardia may occur with bupivacaine; concomitant use of IV verapamil and IV dantrolene may result in cardiovascular collapse; decreases lithium effect and neurotoxicity; decreased clearance with cimetidine; chemically incompatible with solutions of bicarbonate or nafcillin; may be displaced or displace from binding sites, other highly protein-bound drugs such as oral anticoagulants, hydantoins, salicylates, sulfonamides, sulfonylureas.

Guidelines/Precautions

1. May worsen heart failure in patients with poor left ventricular function.
2. Excessive bradycardia, AV block may be treated with isoproterenol, calcium chloride, norepinephrine, atropine, or cardiac pacing.
3. Rapid ventricular rate (because of antegrade conduction) in flutter/fibrillation with Wolff-Parkinson-White syndrome may be treated with procainamide, lidocaine, or DC cardioversion.
4. Use with caution in patients receiving any highly protein-bound drug such as oral anticoagulants, hydantoins, salicylates, sulfonamides, sulfonylureas.
5. Do not chew or divide SR tablets.

Principal Adverse Reactions

Cardiovascular: Hypotension, bradycardia, tachycardia.
Pulmonary: Bronchospasm, laryngospasm.
CNS: Dizziness, headache, seizures.
GI: Nausea, abdominal discomfort.
Allergic: Urticaria, pruritus.

Inhalation
Anesthetics

II

DESFLURANE (SUPRANE)

Use(s): Inhalation anesthesia.
Dosing: Titrate to effect for induction or maintenance of anesthesia.
Elimination: Pulmonary, hepatic, renal.
How Supplied: Volatile liquid.

Pharmacology

Desflurane is a nonflammable fluorinated methyl ethyl ether. It differs from isoflurane by the substitution of a fluorine atom instead of chlorine. It has a vapor pressure of approximately 673 mm Hg at 20° C and boils at 23.5° C. Unlike other volatile anesthetics, desflurane cannot be delivered by standard vaporizers, and requires the use of electrically heated vaporizers and flow meters calibrated in mL/min vapor output. It is less potent than isoflurane, with an MAC in 100% O_2 of 6% atm and in 60% nitrous oxide of 2.8% atm. The blood/gas partition coefficient at 37° C is 0.42. This low solubility in blood means a rapid induction of anesthesia. After 30 min of administration, the ratio of alveolar concentrations to the inspired concentration is 0.9 compared with 0.85 for sevoflurane, 0.99 for nitrous oxide, and 0.73 for isoflurane. Unlike sevoflurane, desflurane may cause coughing and excitation, which may limit the speed of induction. The low tissue solubility of desflurane (fat/blood partition coefficient, 18.7) results in rapid elimination and awakening. After 5 min, the ratio of the alveolar concentration relative to the concentration present at the conclusion of administration is 0.14 compared with 0.22 for isoflurane. Desflurane is very resistant to degradation by soda lime and thus can be used in low-flow or closed systems anesthesia. Compared with isoflurane, desflurane undergoes significantly less metabolism to fluoride and nonvolatile organic fluoride compounds. A 1-MAC-hour does not result in any change in the serum fluoride concentration. Like isoflurane, desflurane causes a moderate increase in $Paco_2$ (approximately 20%), reflecting an increase in the rate of breathing insufficient to offset a decrease in tidal volume. Depression of ventilation reflects a direct depressant effect on the medullary ventilatory center and perhaps peripheral effects on intercostal muscle function. Bronchial smooth muscle relaxation may be produced by a direct effect or indirectly by reductions in afferent nerve traffic or central medullary depression of bronchoconstriction reflexes. Desflurane produces dose-dependent reductions of arterial blood pressure principally because of peripheral vasodilation. Mean arterial pressure is preserved to a greater degree than with equipotent doses of isoflurane. There is little effect on heart rate. Desflurane attenuates baroreceptor reflex responses (tachycardia) to hypotension and vasomotor reflex responses (increased peripheral resistance) to hypovolemia. At equipotent concentrations, desflurane produces less direct decreases in myocardial contractility than isoflurane. Like isoflurane, desflurane does not sensitize the heart to catecholamines. In one study, the dose of submucosally injected epinephrine necessary to produce ventricular cardiac arrhythmias in 50% of patients anesthetized with a 0.8 MAC concentration of desflurane was 6.9 µg/kg compared with an epinephrine dose of 5.7 µg/kg with a 0.7 MAC concentration of isoflurane. Unlike isoflurane, desflurane does not cause coronary artery vasodilation that may lead to coronary artery steal syndrome. Decrease in cerebral metabolic rate is closely linked to cerebral electrical activity. Increased anesthetic concentrations decrease EEG wave frequency and increases voltage with electrical silence at high concentrations. Desflurane, like isoflurane, may produce a dose-related decrease in the amplitude and increase in the latency of cortical components of somatosensory-evoked potentials. The latencies of certain peaks of brain stem auditory-evoked potentials may be increased. Cerebral vasodilation produced by desflurane causes an increase in cerebral blood flow and cerebral blood volume. Elevation of intracranial pressure parallels increase in cerebral blood flow. The increase in cerebral blood flow is attenuated with time and reflects a return of cerebral vascular autoregulation. Hyperventilation of the lungs ($Paco_2 \leq 30$ mm Hg) may not decrease the intracranial pressure. Desflurane has a direct muscle relaxant effect, and potentiation of neuromuscular blocking drugs may involve desensitization of the postjunctional membrane. Desflurane can trigger malignant hyperthermia in susceptible swine.

Pharmacokinetics

Onset of Action: Loss of eyelid reflex (2.5 MAC desflurane over 1–2 min)..

Peak Effect: Dose dependent.

Duration of Action: Emergence time (response to commands) after thiopental sodium for induction and 60% nitrous oxide plus 0.65 MAC desflurane is 8.8 min.

Interaction/Toxicity: Ventilatory and circulatory depressant effects decreased by nitrous oxide substitution; circulatory depressant effects potentiated by arterial hypoxemia, antihypertensives, β-adrenergic antagonists, calcium channel blockers; potentiates depolarizing and nondepolarizing muscle relaxants; MAC decreased by nitrous oxide, clonidine, lithium, ketamine, pancuronium, narcotic agonists, narcotic agonist-antagonist, physostigmine, neostigmine, sedative-hypnotics, chlorpromazine, verapamil, hypothermia, hyponatremia, hypoosmolality, pregnancy, Δ-9-tetrahydrocannabinol; MAC increased by MAO inhibitors, ephedrine, levodopa, chronic ethanol abuse, hypernatremia, hyperthermia, acute cocaine and acute amphetamine ingestion.

Guidelines/Precautions

1. Patients with stenotic lesions of the aortic or mitral valves poorly tolerate changes in blood pressure and systemic vascular resistance.
2. The MAC is highest in the first 6 months of life and is slightly lower in neonates. Beyond adolescence, anesthetic requirements decrease with age so that an 80-year-old patient should require only three fourths the alveolar concentration for anesthesia required for a young adult.
3. Produces dose-related depression of uterine contractility and tone, which can contribute to perioperative blood loss. How-

ever, the uterine response to oxytocic drugs is blocked only at high concentrations (>0.5%).

4. Crosses the placental barrier, and the degree of fetal and neonatal depression (hypotension, hypoxia, acidosis) is directly proportional to the depth and duration of maternal anesthesia.

5. Changes in mental function may persist beyond the period of anesthetic administration and the immediate postoperative period. There may be altered psychomotor performance and driving skills.

6. Contraindicated in patients with known or suspected genetic susceptibility to malignant hyperthermia.

7. Abrupt onset of malignant hyperthermia may be triggered by desflurane. Early premonitory signs include muscle rigidity, especially jaw muscles, tachycardia and tachypnea unresponsive to increased depth of anesthesia, evidence of increased oxygen consumption and carbon dioxide production (change in color and increased temperature of the carbon dioxide absorber), rising body temperature, and metabolic acidosis.

Principal Adverse Reactions

Cardiovascular: Hypotension, arrhythmias.
Pulmonary: Respiratory depression, apnea.
CNS: Dizziness, euphoria, increased cerebral blood flow and intracranial pressure.
GI/Hepatic: Nausea, vomiting, ileus, hepatic dysfunction.
Metabolic: Malignant hyperthermia.

ENFLURANE (ETHRANE)

Use(s): Inhalation anesthesia.
Dosing: Titrate to effect for induction or maintenance of anesthesia.
Elimination: Pulmonary, hepatic, renal.
How Supplied: Volatile liquid, 125 mL, 250 mL.

Pharmacology

Enflurane is a nonflammable fluorinated ethyl methyl ether. It has a vapor pressure of approximately 175 mm Hg at 20° C and boils at 56.5° C. In this respect it is similar to other volatile anesthetics and can be delivered by standard vaporizers. It is less potent than isoflurane, with an MAC in 100% O_2 of 1.7% atm and in 70% nitrous oxide of 0.6% atm. The blood/gas partition coefficient at 37° C is 1.91. The intermediate solubility in blood combined with a high potency means a rapid induction of anesthesia. After 30 min of administration, the ratios of alveolar concentrations to the inspired concentration is 0.65 compared with 0.99 for nitrous oxide and 0.73 for isoflurane. The intermediate tissue solubility of enflurane (fat/blood partition coefficient, 36.0) results in rapid elimination and awakening. After 5 min, the ratio of the alveolar concentration relative to the concentration present at the conclusion of administration is 0.14 compared with 0.22 for isoflurane. Enflurane is slowly metabolized by the hepatic mixed function oxidase system. Biotransformation releases fluoride ions by oxidative dehalogenation. Peak plasma fluoride concentrations after a 2.5-MAC-hour exposure to enflurane are about 20 μmol/L, which is approximately one third the level considered to be potentially nephrotoxic. Enflurane is resistant to degradation by soda lime and thus can be used in low-flow or closed systems anesthesia. Like isoflurane, enflurane causes a moderate increase in Pa_{CO_2} (approximately 20%), reflecting an increase in the rate of breathing insufficient to offset a decrease in tidal volume. Depression of ventilation reflects a direct depressant effect on the medullary ventilatory center and perhaps peripheral effects on intercostal muscle function. Bronchial smooth muscle relaxation may be produced by a direct effect or indirectly by reductions in afferent nerve traffic or central medullary depression of bronchoconstriction reflexes. Enflurane inhibits the hypoxic pulmonary vasoconstrictor (HPV) response in a dose-related manner. It has little or no effect on pulmonary vascular smooth muscle. Enflurane produces dose-dependent reductions of arterial blood pressure in part or whole, a consequence of decreases in myocardial contractility and cardiac output. It produces dose-dependent elevations in heart rate. Enflurane attenuates baroreceptor reflex responses (tachycardia) to hypotension and vasomotor reflex responses (increased peripheral resistance) to hypovolemia. Like isoflurane, enflurane does not sensitize the heart to catecholamines. In one study, the dose of submucosally injected epinephrine necessary to produce ventricular cardiac arrhythmias in 50% of patients anesthetized with a 1.25 MAC concentration of enflurane was 3.5 μg/kg compared with 1.5 μg/kg for halothane and 6.5 μg/kg for isoflurane. Unlike isoflurane, enflurane does not cause coronary artery vasodilation that may lead to coronary artery steal syndrome. Decrease in cerebral metabolic rate is closely linked to cerebral electrical activity. Increased anesthetic concentrations decrease EEG wave frequency and increase voltage. Electrical silence does not occur, but a high-voltage repetitive-spiking activity may be produced. This activity may be attenuated or abolished by decreasing the enflurane dose or increasing the arterial carbon dioxide partial pressure ($PaCO_2$ >30 mm Hg). Enflurane does not enhance preexisting epileptic foci, with the possible exceptions being certain types of myoclonic epilepsy and photosensitive epilepsy. Enflurane compared with isoflurane or halothane produces the greatest dose-related decrease in the amplitude and increase in the latency of cortical components of somatosensory-evoked potentials. The latencies of certain peaks of brain stem auditory-evoked potentials may be increased. Cerebral vasodilation produced by enflurane causes an increase in cerebral blood flow and cerebral blood volume. Elevation of intracranial pressure parallels increase in cerebral blood flow. Unlike isoflurane or halothane, hyperventilation does not attenuate such increase but, on the contrary, increases the risk of seizure activity, which could lead to an elevation in cerebral metabolic oxygen requirements, carbon dioxide production, increased cerebral blood flow, and increased intracranial pressure. Enflurane increases both the rate of production and resistance to reabsorption of cerebrospinal fluid, which may contribute to sustained increases in intracranial pressure associated with administration of this anesthetic. Enflurane has a direct muscle relaxant effect, and potentiation of neuromuscular blocking drugs may involve desensitization of the postjunctional membrane. Enflurane can trigger malignant hyperthermia in susceptible swine.

Pharmacokinetics

Onset of Action: Loss of eyelid reflex (2.4 MAC enflurane plus 66% N_2O): 2.9 min.

Peak Effect: Surgical anesthesia: 2%–4.5% produces anesthesia in 7–10 min.

Duration of Action: Emergence time (response to commands) after thiopental for induction and 66% nitrous oxide plus 0.9 MAC enflurane: 15.1 min.

Interaction/Toxicity: Ventilatory and circulatory depressant effects decreased by nitrous oxide substitution: circulatory depressant effects potentiated by arterial hypoxemia, antihypertensives, β-adrenergic antagonists, calcium channel blockers; isoniazid increases defluorination of enflurane in genetically susceptible patients (e.g., rapid acetylators); potentiates depolarizing and nondepolarizing muscle relaxants; MAC decreased by nitrous oxide, clonidine, lithium, ketamine, pancuronium, narcotic agonists, narcotic agonist-antagonist, physostigmine, neostigmine, sedative-hypnotics, chlorpromazine, verapamil, hypothermia, hyponatremia, hypoosmolality, pregnancy, Δ-9-tetrahydrocannabinol; MAC increased by MAO inhibitors, ephedrine, levo-dopa, chronic ethanol abuse, hypernatremia, hyperthermia, acute cocaine and acute amphetamine ingestion.

Guidelines/Precautions

1. Patients with stenotic lesions of the aortic or mitral valves poorly tolerate changes in blood pressure and systemic vascular resistance.
2. The MAC is highest in the first 6 months of life and is slightly lower in neonates. Beyond adolescence, anesthetic requirements decrease with age, so that an 80-year-old patient should require only three fourths the alveolar concentration for anesthesia required for a young adult.
3. Produces dose-related depression of uterine contractility and tone that can contribute to perioperative blood loss. However, the uterine response to oxytocic drugs is blocked only at high concentrations (>1.0%).
4. Crosses the placental barrier, and the degree of fetal and neonatal depression (hypotension, hypoxia, acidosis) is directly proportional to the depth and duration of maternal anesthesia.
5. Changes in mental function may persist beyond the period of anesthetic administration and the immediate postoperative period. There may be altered psychomotor performance and driving skills.
6. Contraindicated in patients with seizure disorders and known or suspected genetic susceptibility to malignant hyperthermia.
7. Abrupt onset of malignant hyperthermia may be triggered by enflurane. Early premonitory signs include muscle rigidity, especially jaw muscles, tachycardia and tachypnea unresponsive to increased depth of anesthesia, evidence of increased

oxygen consumption and carbon dioxide production, (change in color and increased temperature of the carbon dioxide absorber), rising body temperature, and metabolic acidosis.

Principal Adverse Reactions

Cardiovascular: Hypotension, arrhythmias.
Pulmonary: Respiratory depression, apnea.
CNS: Seizures, dizziness, euphoria, increased cerebral blood flow and intracranial pressure.
GI: Nausea, vomiting, hepatic dysfunction.
GU: Renal dysfunction, renal failure.
Musculoskeletal: Motor activity of various muscle groups.
Metabolic: Malignant hyperthermia, glucose elevation.

HALOTHANE (FLUOTHANE)

Use(s): Inhalation anesthesia.
Dosing: Titrate to effect for induction or maintenance of anesthesia.
Elimination: Pulmonary, hepatic, renal.
How Supplied: Volatile liquid: 125 mL, 250 mL.

Pharmacology

A nonflammable halogenated alkene, halothane is 2-bromo-2-chloro-1,1,1-trifluoroethane. It has a vapor pressure of approximately 241 mm Hg at 20° and boils at 50.2° C. In this way, it is similar to other volatile anesthetics and can be delivered by standard vaporizers. It is more potent than isoflurane, with an MAC in 100% O_2 of 0.77% atm and in 66% nitrous oxide of 0.29% atm. The blood/gas partition coefficient at 37° C is 2.3. The intermediate solubility in blood, combined with a high potency, permits rapid onset and recovery from anesthesia. After 30 min of administration, the ratio of alveolar concentration to the inspired concentration in adults is 0.58 compared with 0.99 for nitrous oxide and 0.73 for isoflurane. The alveolar rate of rise of halothane is more rapid in children, with alveolar concentration to the inspired concentration ratio of 0.8 after 30 min. This probably results from the greater ventilation and perfusion per kg of tissue in children.

and the fact that the increased perfusion is devoted mainly in the vessel-rich group. After the first few minutes of emergence, with alveolar concentration <0.01 MAC, rapid decline of alveolar concentrations depends more on metabolism and less on blood solubility. The intermediate tissue solubility (fat/blood partition coefficient, 60.0) and considerable metabolism of halothane result in rapid elimination and awakening. After 5 min, the ratios of the alveolar concentration relative to the concentration present at the conclusion of administration is 0.25 compared with 0.22 for isoflurane. Halothane is susceptible to decomposition to hydrochloric acid, hydrobromic acid, chloride, bromide, and phosgene. For this reason, it is stored in amber-colored bottles, and thymol is added as a preservative to prevent spontaneous oxidative decomposition. Thymol that remains in vaporizers after vaporization of halothane can cause vaporizer turnstiles or temperature-compensating devices to malfunction. Halothane does not decompose in contact with warm soda lime and thus can be used in low-flow or closed systems anesthesia. When moisture is present, the vapor attacks aluminium, brass, and lead but not copper. Rubber, some plastics, and similar materials are soluble in halothane (rubber/gas partition coefficient of 120 for halothane compared with 62 for isoflurane, 74 for enflurane, and 1.2 for nitrous oxide) and will deteriorate rapidly in contact with halothane liquid or vapor. Like isoflurane, halothane causes a moderate increase in $Paco_2$ (approximately 20%), reflecting an increase in the rate of breathing insufficient to offset a decrease in tidal volume. Depression of ventilation reflects a direct depressant effect on the medullary ventilatory center and perhaps peripheral effects on intercostal muscle function. Bronchial smooth muscle relaxation may be produced by a direct effect or indirectly by reductions in afferent nerve traffic or central medullary depression of bronchoconstriction reflexes. Halothane inhibits the HPV response at inspired concentrations of ≥3%. It has little or no effect on pulmonary vascular smooth muscle. Halothane produces dose-dependent reductions of arterial blood pressure in part or whole, a consequence of decreases in myocardial contractility and cardiac output. Halothane frequently decreases heart rate (reversible with atropine) and may slow the conduction of cardiac impulses through the AV node and His-Purkinje system. This increases the likelihood of cardiac arrhythmias because of a reentry mechanism. Junctional rhythm leading to reductions of blood pressure may occur during administration of halothane and most likely reflects suppression of sinus node activity. Halothane attenuates baroreceptor reflex responses (tachycardia) to hypotension and vasomotor reflex responses (increased peripheral resistance) to hypovolemia. It sensitizes the myocardium to the action of epinephrine and norepinephrine; the combination may cause serious cardiac arrhythmias. In one study, the dose of submucosally injected epinephrine necessary to produce ventricular cardiac arrhythmias in 50% of patients anesthetized with a 1.25 MAC concentration of halothane was 1.5 μg/kg compared with 3.5 μg/kg for enflurane and 6.5 μg/kg for isoflurane. In contrast to adults, children tolerate higher doses of SC epinephrine (7.8–10 μg/kg) injected with or without lidocaine during halothane anesthesia. Unlike isoflurane, halothane does not cause coronary artery vasodilation that may lead to coronary artery steal syndrome. Decrease in cerebral metabolic rate is closely linked to cerebral electrical activity. Increased anesthetic concentrations decrease EEG wave frequency and increase voltage with electrical silence at high concentrations (3.5 MAC). Halothane, like isoflurane or enflurane but to a lesser degree, may produce a dose-related decrease in the amplitude and increase in the latency of cortical components of somatosensory-evoked potentials. The latencies of certain peaks of brain stem auditory-evoked potentials may be increased. Cerebral vasodilation and increase in cerebral blood flow and cerebral blood volume produced by halothane are greater than those produced by isoflurane or enflurane (200% increase in cerebral blood flow at 1.1 MAC of halothane compared with 30%–50% increase with enflurane and no change with isoflurane). Elevation of intracranial pressure parallels the increase in cerebral blood flow. The increase in cerebral blood flow is attenuated with time (within 2 hr for halothane) and reflects a return of cerebral vascular autoregulation. Hyperventilation of the lungs (Pa_{CO_2} ≤30 mm Hg) before introduction of halothane opposes the increase in intracranial pressure. Halothane decreases the rate of cerebrospinal fluid production but increases resistance to reabsorption. The increase in cerebrospinal fluid pressure returns to normal with time. Halothane has a direct muscle relaxant effect, and potentiation of neuromuscular blocking drugs may involve desensitization of the postjunctional membrane. Halothane can trigger malignant hyperthermia in susceptible swine.

Pharmacokinetics

Onset of Action: Dose dependent.
Peak Effect: Dose dependent. Decrease in intellectual function: 2 days.
Duration of Action: Dose dependent. Decrease in intellectual function: 8 days.
Interaction/Toxicity: Ventilatory and circulatory depressant effects decreased by nitrous oxide substitution; circulatory depressant effects potentiated by arterial hypoxemia, antihypertensives, β-adrenergic antagonists, calcium channel blockers; potentiates depolarizing and nondepolarizing muscle relaxants; MAC decreased by nitrous oxide, clonidine, lithium, ketamine, pancuronium, narcotic agonists, narcotic agonist-antagonist, physostigmine, neostigmine, sedative-hypnotics, chlorpromazine, verapamil, hypothermia, hyponatremia, hypoosmolality, pregnancy, Δ-9-tetrahydrocannabinol; MAC increased by MAO inhibitors, cocaine, ephedrine, levodopa, chronic ethanol abuse, hypernatremia, hyperthermia.

Guidelines/Precautions

1. Patients with stenotic lesions of the aortic or mitral valves poorly tolerate changes in blood pressure and systemic vascular resistance.
2. The MAC is highest in the first 6 mo of life and is slightly lower in neonates. Beyond adolescence, anesthetic requirements decrease with age so that an 80-year-old patient should require only three fourths the alveolar concentration for anesthesia required for a young adult.
3. Halothane is not recommended for obstetric anesthesia except when uterine relaxation is required. It is a potent uterine relaxant and can contribute to perioperative blood loss. However, the uterine response to oxytocic drugs is blocked only at concentrations >0.25%–0.5%.
4. Crosses the placental barrier; the degree of fetal and neonatal depression (hypotension, hypoxia, acidosis) is directly proportional to the depth and duration of maternal anesthesia.
5. Halothane administration has been associated with hepatic dysfunction. There may be two types: one characterized by transient elevations in serum levels of liver transaminase enzymes (20%–25% of patients) and the other fulminant hepatic

failure (1:7000–1:30,000). Patients at particular risk appear to be middle-aged obese women with previous closely spaced halothane administration.

6. Changes in mental function may persist beyond the period of anesthetic administration and the immediate postoperative period. There may be altered psychomotor performance and driving skills.

7. Contraindicated in patients with known or suspected genetic susceptibility to malignant hyperthermia.

8. Abrupt onset of malignant hyperthermia may be triggered by halothane. Early premonitory signs include muscle rigidity, especially jaw muscles, tachycardia and tachypnea unresponsive to increased depth of anesthesia, evidence of increased oxygen consumption and carbon dioxide production (change in color and increased temperature of the carbon dioxide absorber), rising body temperature and metabolic acidosis.

Principal Adverse Reactions

Cardiovascular: Hypotension, bradycardia, arrhythmias.
Pulmonary: Respiratory depression, apnea.
CNS: Dizziness, euphoria, increased cerebral blood flow and intracranial pressure.
GI/Hepatic: Nausea, vomiting, ileus, hepatic dysfunction, fulminant hepatic failure.
Metabolic: Malignant hyperthermia.

ISOFLURANE (FORANE)

Use(s): Inhalation anesthesia.
Dosing: Titrate to effect for induction or maintenance of anesthesia.
Elimination: Pulmonary, hepatic, renal.
How Supplied: Volatile liquid, 100 mL.

Pharmacology

Isoflurane is a nonflammable halogenated methyl ethyl ether. It has a vapor pressure of approximately 238 mm Hg at 20° C and boils at 48.5° C (760 mm Hg atmospheric pressure). In this respect it is similar to other volatile anesthetics and can be delivered by standard vaporizers. It has an MAC in 100% O_2 of 1.15% atm and in 70% nitrous oxide of 0.5% atm. The blood/gas partition coefficient is 1.4. This intermediate solubility in blood combined with a high potency means a rapid induction of anesthesia. After 30 min of administration, the ratio of alveolar concentrations to the inspired concentration is 0.73. The intermediate tissue solubility of isoflurane (fat/blood partition coefficient, 45.0) results in rapid elimination and awakening. After 5 min, the ratio of the alveolar concentration relative to the concentration present at the conclusion of administration is 0.22 for isoflurane. Isoflurane is resistant to degradation by soda lime and thus can be used in low-flow or closed systems anesthesia. Isoflurane causes a moderate increase in Pa_{CO_2} (approximately 20%), reflecting an increase in the rate of breathing insufficient to offset a decrease in tidal volume. Unlike other inhaled anesthetics, >1 MAC concentration, isoflurane does not produce a further increase in the rate of breathing. Depression of ventilation reflects a direct depressant effect on the medullary ventilatory center and perhaps peripheral effects on intercostal muscle function. Bronchial smooth muscle relaxation may be produced by a direct effect or indirectly by reductions in afferent nerve traffic or central medullary depression of bronchoconstriction reflexes. Isoflurane inhibits the HPV response in a dose-related manner. It has little or no effect on pulmonary vascular smooth muscle. Isoflurane produces dose-dependent reductions of arterial blood pressure caused principally by peripheral vasodilation. It elevates heart rate 20% above awake levels and independent of doses >1 MAC. Heart rate increases are more likely to occur in young than elderly patients or neonates and may be accentuated by the presence of other drugs (atropine, meperidine, pancuronium) that independently increase heart rate. Depression of baroreceptor reflex responses (tachycardia) to hypotension and vasomotor reflex responses (increased peripheral resistance) to hypovolemia is less pronounced with isoflurane compared with halothane or enflurane. Decreases in stroke volume are offset by an increase in heart rate such that cardiac output is unchanged. At equipotent concentrations, isoflurane and desflurane produce equivalent direct decreases in myocardial contractility. Isoflurane does not sensitize the heart to catecholamines. In one study, the dose of submucosally injected epinephrine necessary to produce ventricular cardiac arrhythmias in 50% of patients anesthetized with a 1.25 MAC concentration of isoflurane was 6.5 μg/kg compared with 1.5 μg/kg for halothane and 3.5 μg/kg for enflurane. It causes coronary artery vasodilation that may lead to coronary artery steal syndrome. However, there is no evidence of different outcomes for coronary revascularization operations in patients anesthetized primarily with isoflurane compared with enflurane, halothane, or sufentanil. Isoflurane undergoes minimal metabolism, reflecting its chemical stability and low solubility in tissues. Trifluoroacetic acid is the principal organic fluoride metabolite. The minimal changes in plasma concentrations of fluoride resulting from metabolism of isoflurane plus the absence of reductive metabolism render nephrotoxicity or hepatotoxicity after administration of isoflurane unlikely. Decrease in cerebral metabolic rate is closely linked to cerebral electrical activity. Increased anesthetic concentrations decrease EEG wave frequency and increase voltage with electrical silence at high concentrations. Isoflurane may produce a dose-related decrease in the amplitude and increase in the latency of cortical components of somatosensory-evoked potentials. The latencies of certain peaks of brain stem auditory-evoked potentials may be increased. At 1.1 MAC isoflurane, cerebral vasodilation is minimal or unchanged. Increased concentrations cause an increase in cerebral blood flow and cerebral blood volume. Elevation of intracranial pressure parallels increase in cerebral blood flow. The increase in cerebral blood flow is attenuated with time and reflects a return of cerebral vascular autoregulation. Hyperventilation of the lungs ($Paco_2 \leq 30$ mm Hg) simultaneous with introduction of isoflurane opposes the increase in intracranial pressure. Isoflurane does not alter production of cerebrospinal fluid and at the same time decreases resistance to its reabsorption. This is consistent with minimal increases in intracranial pressure observed. Isoflurane has a direct muscle relaxant effect and potentiation of neuromuscular blocking drugs may involve desensitization of the postjunctional membrane. Isoflurane can trigger malignant hyperthermia in susceptible swine.

Pharmacokinetics

Onset of Action: Few minutes (dose dependent).
Peak Effect: Surgical anesthesia: 1.5%–3.0% produces anesthesia in 7–10 min.

Duration of Action: Emergence time (response to commands) after thiopental for induction and 60% nitrous oxide plus 0.65 MAC: 15.6 min.

Interaction/Toxicity: Ventilatory and circulatory depressant effects decreased by nitrous oxide substitution; circulatory depressant effects potentiated by arterial hypoxemia, antihypertensives, β-adrenergic antagonists, calcium channel blockers; potentiates depolarizing and nondepolarizing muscle relaxants; MAC decreased by nitrous oxide, clonidine, lithium, ketamine, pancuronium, narcotic agonists, narcotic agonist-antagonist, physostigmine, neostigmine, sedative-hypnotics, chlorpromazine, verapamil, hypothermia, hyponatremia, hypoosmolality, pregnancy, Δ-9-tetrahydrocannabinol; MAC increased by MAO inhibitors, ephedrine, levodopa, chronic ethanol abuse, hypernatremia, hyperthermia, acute cocaine and acute amphetamine ingestion.

Guidelines/Precautions

1. Patients with stenotic lesions of the aortic or mitral valves poorly tolerate changes in blood pressure and systemic vascular resistance
2. The MAC is highest in the first 6 months of life and is slightly lower in neonates. Beyond adolescence, anesthetic requirements decrease with age so that an 80-year-old patient should require only three fourths the alveolar concentration for anesthesia required for a young adult.
3. Produces dose-related depression of uterine contractility and tone, which can contribute to perioperative blood loss. However, the uterine response to oxytocic drugs is blocked only at high concentrations ($>0.75\%$).
4. Crosses the placental barrier; the degree of fetal and neonatal depression (hypotension, hypoxia, acidosis) is directly proportional to the depth and duration of maternal anesthesia.
5. Changes in mental function may persist beyond the period of anesthetic administration and the immediate postoperative period. There may be altered psychomotor performance and driving skills.
6. Contraindicated in patients with known or suspected genetic susceptibility to malignant hyperthermia.
7. Abrupt onset of malignant hyperthermia may be triggered by isoflurane. Early premonitory signs include muscle rigidity,

especially jaw muscles, tachycardia and tachypnea unresponsive to increased depth of anesthesia, evidence of increased
oxygen consumption and carbon dioxide production (change
in color and increased temperature of the carbon dioxide absorber), rising body temperature and metabolic acidosis.

Principal Adverse Reactions

Cardiovascular: Hypotension, tachycardia, arrhythmias, coro-
nary artery steal.
Pulmonary: Respiratory depression, apnea.
CNS: Dizziness, euphoria, increased cerebral blood flow and in-
tracranial pressure.
GI/Hepatic: Nausea, vomiting, ileus, hepatic dysfunction.
Metabolic: Malignant hyperthermia, glucose elevation.

NITROUS OXIDE (NITROUS OXIDE)

Use(s): Inhalation analgesic, supplementation of anesthesia.
Dosing: Titrate to effect for analgesia, induction, or maintenance
of anesthesia.
Elimination: Pulmonary, renal, GI tract.
How Supplied: Blue cylinders.

Pharmacology

A strong analgesic and weak anesthetic usually used in combination with other anesthetics. Although nitrous oxide is nonflammable, it will support combustion. It has a vapor pressure of approximately 39,000 mm Hg at 20° C and boils at $-88.0°$ C. It has an
MAC with oxygen of 104% atm. The blood/gas partition coefficient for nitrous oxide is 0.47 compared with 1.4 for isoflurane.
This low solubility in blood means a rapid induction of anesthesia. After 30 min of administration, the ratio of alveolar concentration to the inspired concentration is 0.99 compared with 0.73
for isoflurane. The very low tissue solubility of nitrous oxide (fat/
blood partition coefficient 2.3 compared with fat/blood partition
coefficient 45.0 for isoflurane) results in rapid elimination and
awakening. After 5 min, the ratio of the alveolar concentration
relative to the concentration present at the conclusion of adminis-

tration is 0.14 compared with 0.22 for isoflurane. Administration of high concentrations of a rapidly absorbed first gas will facilitate the rate of rise in alveolar concentration of a concomitantly administered second gas, a phenomenon called the second gas effect. This effect is most pronounced when nitrous oxide is combined with a volatile anesthetic. Nitrous oxide is resistant to degradation by soda lime and thus can be used in low-flow or closed systems anesthesia. Unlike the other inhaled anesthetics, nitrous oxide does not increase the Pa_{CO_2}. It increases the rate of breathing more than other inhaled anesthetics. Depression of ventilation occurs at high concentrations (>50%) and reflects a direct depressant effect on the medullary ventilatory center and perhaps peripheral effects on intercostal muscle function. Like other inhaled anesthetics, nitrous oxide decreases functional residual capacity. Bronchial smooth muscle relaxation may be produced by a direct effect or indirectly by reductions in afferent nerve traffic or central medullary depression of bronchoconstriction reflexes. Nitrous oxide does not inhibit the HPV response. It may produce increases in pulmonary vascular resistance that are exaggerated in patients with preexisting pulmonary hypertension. Alone in a 40% concentration, nitrous oxide directly depresses the myocardium. When it is given to patients with heart disease, particularly in combination with opioids, it will cause hypotension and a decrease in cardiac output. Combined with other inhaled anesthetics (e.g., desflurane, enflurane, halothane, isoflurane, sevoflurane), nitrous oxide is sympathomimetic and has mild cardiac depressant effects. There is decreased cardiac output, increased systemic vascular resistance, and increased arterial pressure. Reduction of concentration and substitution of some of the required volatile anesthetic with nitrous oxide lead to less depression of the circulation at a given MAC level than with either agent alone. There is little effect on heart rate. Nitrous oxide attenuates baroreceptor reflex responses (tachycardia) to hypotension and vasomotor reflex responses (increased peripheral resistance) to hypovolemia. Nitrous oxide enhances isoflurane-induced coronary artery vasodilation that may lead to coronary artery steal syndrome. However, 50% nitrous oxide plus a low concentration of isoflurane (about 0.4 MAC) administered to patients with coronary artery disease improves tolerance to pacing-induced myocardial ischemia. Nitrous oxide probably is not metabolized by human tissue. An estimated

0.04% undergoes reductive metabolism to nitrogen in the GI tract. Anaerobic bacteria such as *Pseudomonas* are responsible for this reductive metabolism. Reductive products of some nitrogen compounds include free radicals that could produce toxic effects on cells. The potential toxic role of these metabolites, however, remains undocumented. Nitrous oxide inhibits methionine synthetase activity by oxidizing the cobalt atom in vitamin B_{12} from an active to an inactive state. Inhibition of enzyme activity results in decreased availability of tetrahydrofolate, which is necessary for the synthesis of DNA. Interference with DNA synthesis could manifest as spontaneous abortions, congenital anomalies, depression of bone marrow function, and polyneuropathy resembling pernicious anemia in individuals chronically exposed to high concentrations of nitrous oxide. Decrease in cerebral metabolic rate is closely linked to cerebral electrical activity. Increased anesthetic concentrations decrease EEG wave frequency and increase voltage with electrical silence at high concentrations. Nitrous oxide may produce greater attenuations of somatosensory-evoked potentials than low concentrations of enflurane or isoflurane. Cortical responses are more affected than subcortical responses. Nitrous oxide can increase the latency and decrease amplitude of cortical components of visual and auditory evoked potentials. To a modest degree, cerebral vasodilation produced by nitrous oxide causes an increase in cerebral blood flow and cerebral blood volume. Elevation of intracranial pressure parallels increase in cerebral blood flow. The increase in cerebral blood flow is attenuated with time and reflects a return of cerebral vascular autoregulation. Hyperventilation of the lungs ($Paco_2 \leq 30$ mm Hg) opposes the increase in intracranial pressure. Nitrous oxide does not relax skeletal muscles and in doses that exceed 1 MAC may produce skeletal muscle rigidity. It does not have significant effects on uterine contractility. Nitrous oxide compared with volatile anesthetics is a weak trigger for malignant hyperthermia.

Pharmacokinetics

Onset of Action: Few minutes (dose dependent).
Peak Effect: Dose dependent.
Duration of Action: Varies (dose dependent). Emergence time (response to commands) after thiopental for induction and 60% nitrous oxide plus 0.65 MAC isoflurane: 15.6 min. Memory impairment: ≥ 24 hr.

Interaction/Toxicity: Ventilatory depressant effects potentiated by volatile anesthetics; circulatory depressant effects potentiated by arterial hypoxemia, volatile anesthetics, antihypertensives, β-adrenergic antagonists, calcium channel blockers; increases toxic effects of methotrexate, e.g., leukopenia; facilitates uptake of other inhalation anesthetics (second gas effect); reduces requirements for volatile anesthetics approximately equal to 1% of the MAC value for each volume-percent alveolar nitrous oxide concentration.

Guidelines/Precautions

1. The chief danger in the use of nitrous oxide is hypoxia; at least 30% oxygen should be used.
2. Nitrous oxide diffuses into air-containing cavities 34 times faster than nitrogen can leave, causing potentially dangerous pressure accumulation (e.g., middle ear abnormalities, bowel obstruction, pneumothorax). Nitrous oxide (to a greater extent than other gases) diffuses into air-inflated endotracheal tube cuffs and increases intracuff volume and pressure that may result in significant glottic or subglottic trauma. Therefore, during general anesthesia, intracuff volume and pressure should be periodically readjusted.
3. During the first 5–10 min of recovery from anesthesia, the outpouring of large volumes of nitrous oxide may displace alveolar oxygen and produce diffusion hypoxia. Displacement of alveolar carbon dioxide may decrease respiratory drive and hence ventilation. It is prudent to administer 100% oxygen at this critical time of recovery.
4. In healthy patients undergoing surgery, megaloblastic bone marrow changes may be seen after about 12 hr of exposure to 50% nitrous oxide and earlier in seriously ill patients. These changes may be preventable by pretreating patients with large doses of folinic acid. Folinic acid is converted to tetrahydrofolate, which is necessary for the synthesis of DNA.
5. An increased risk of renal and hepatic diseases has been reported in dental personnel who work in areas where nitrous oxide is used. Nitrous oxide may precipitate neurologic disease in patients with unrecognized vitamin B_{12} deficiency.
6. Patients with stenotic lesions of the aortic or mitral valves poorly tolerate changes in blood pressure and systemic vascular resistance.

7. Crosses the placental barrier; the degree of fetal and neonatal depression (hypotension, hypoxia, acidosis) is directly proportional to the depth and duration of maternal anesthesia.

8. The newborn with or without preexisting pulmonary hypertension may be uniquely vulnerable to the pulmonary vascular constricting effects of nitrous oxide. In patients with congenital heart disease, these increases in pulmonary vascular resistance may increase the magnitude of right-to-left intracardiac shunting of blood and further jeopardize arterial oxygenation.

9. Changes in mental function may persist beyond the period of anesthetic administration and the immediate postoperative period. There may be altered psychomotor performance and driving skills.

10. Use only with extreme caution and vigilant monitoring in patients with known or suspected genetic susceptibility to malignant hyperthermia.

11. Abrupt onset of malignant hyperthermia may be triggered by nitrous oxide. Early premonitory signs include muscle rigidity, especially jaw muscles, tachycardia and tachypnea unresponsive to increased depth of anesthesia, evidence of increased oxygen consumption and carbon dioxide production (change in color and increased temperature of the carbon dioxide absorber), rising body temperature and metabolic acidosis.

Principal Adverse Reactions

Cardiovascular: Hypotension, arrhythmias.
Pulmonary: Respiratory depression, apnea, diffusion hypoxia.
CNS: Dizziness, euphoria, increased cerebral blood flow and intracranial pressure, peripheral neuropathy, subacute combined degeneration of the spinal cord (with chronic abuse and gross exposure).
GI/Hepatic: Nausea, vomiting, ileus.
Hematologic: Megaloblastic anemia, bone marrow depression.
Metabolic: Malignant hyperthermia.

SEVOFLURANE (SEVOFLURANE)

Use(s): Inhalation anesthesia.
Dosing: Titrate to effect for induction or maintenance of anesthesia.
Elimination: Pulmonary, hepatic, renal.
How Supplied: Volatile liquid.

Pharmacology

Sevoflurane is a nonflammable fluorinated isopropyl ether. It has a vapor pressure of approximately 162 mm Hg at 20° C and boils at 58.5° C. In this respect it is similar to other volatile anesthetics and can be delivered by standard vaporizers. It is less potent than isoflurane, with an MAC in 100% O_2 of 1.71% atm and in 63.5% nitrous oxide of 0.66% atm. The blood/gas partition coefficient at 37° C is 0.59. This low solubility in blood means a rapid induction of anesthesia. Sevoflurane is less of an irritant to the upper respiratory tract than desflurane, causing less coughing and laryngospasm on induction. After 30 min of administration, the ratio of alveolar concentrations to the inspired concentration is 0.85 compared with 0.9 for desflurane, 0.99 for nitrous oxide, and 0.73 for isoflurane. The low tissue solubility of servoflurane (fat/blood partition coefficient, 53.4) results in rapid elimination and awakening. After 5 min, the ratio of the alveolar concentration relative to the concentration present at the conclusion of administration is 0.16 compared with 0.22 for isoflurane. Sevoflurane undergoes temperature-dependent degradation by soda lime and baralyme and thus cannot be used in low-flow or closed systems anesthesia. Like isoflurane, sevoflurane causes a moderate increase in $Paco_2$ (approximately 20%) reflecting an increase in the rate of breathing insufficient to offset a decrease in tidal volume. Depression of ventilation reflects a direct depressant effect on the medullary ventilatory center and perhaps peripheral effects on intercostal muscle function. Bronchial smooth muscle relaxation may be produced by a direct effect or indirectly by reductions in afferent nerve traffic or central medullary depression of bronchoconstriction reflexes. Sevoflurane produces dose-dependent reductions of arterial blood pressure caused principally by peripheral vasodilation. There is little effect on heart rate. Sevoflurane attenuates baroreceptor reflex responses (tachycardia) to hypotension and vasomotor reflex responses (increased peripheral resistance) to hypovolemia. At equipotent concentrations, sevoflurane and isoflurane produce equivalent direct decreases in myocardial contractility. Like isoflurane, sevoflurane does not sensitize the heart to catecholamines. The arrhythmogenic threshold is intermediate between enflurane and isoflurane. In one study, the dose of submucosally injected epinephrine necessary to produce ventricular cardiac arrhythmias in 50% of patients anesthetized with a 1.3 MAC concentration of sevoflurane was 8.57 μg/kg compared with 5.17 μg/kg for enflurane and 9.81 μg/kg for isoflurane. Unlike isoflurane, sevoflurane may not cause coronary artery vasodilation that may lead to coronary artery steal syndrome. Sevoflurane undergoes oxidative metabolism in the liver, with a serum fluoride concentration of approximately 22 μmol/L after a 1-MAC-hour exposure. The magnitude of sevoflurane metabolism resembles that of enflurane (peak plasma fluoride concentrations after a 2.5-MAC-hour exposure to enflurane are about 20 μmol/L). Decrease in cerebral metabolic rate is closely linked to cerebral electrical activity. Increased anesthetic concentrations decrease EEG wave frequency and increase voltage with electrical silence at high concentrations. Sevoflurane like isoflurane may produce a dose-related decrease in the amplitude and increase in the latency of cortical components of visual and auditory-evoked potentials. Cerebral vasodilation produced by sevoflurane causes an increase in cerebral blood flow and cerebral blood volume. Elevation of intracranial pressure parallels increase in cerebral blood flow. The increase in cerebral blood flow is attenuated with time and reflects a return of cerebral vascular autoregulation. Hyperventilation of the lungs ($Pa_{CO_2} \leq 30$ mm Hg) opposes the increase in intracranial pressure. Sevoflurane has a direct muscle relaxant effect, and potentiation of neuromuscular blocking drugs may involve desensitization of the postjunctional membrane. Sevoflurane can trigger malignant hyperthermia in susceptible swine.

Pharmacokinetics

Onset of Action: Loss of eyelid reflex (1.8 MAC sevoflurane plus 66% nitrous oxide): 1.6 min.
Peak Effect: Dose dependent.

Duration of Action: Emergence time (response to commands) after thiopental for induction and 66% nitrous oxide plus 0.9 MAC sevoflurane: 14.3 min.

Interaction/Toxicity: Ventilatory and circulatory depressant effects decreased by nitrous oxide substitution; circulatory depressant effects potentiated by arterial hypoxemia, antihypertensives, β-adrenergic antagonists, calcium channel blockers; potentiates depolarizing and nondepolarizing muscle relaxants; MAC decreased by nitrous oxide, clonidine, lithium, ketamine, pancuronium, narcotic agonists, narcotic agonist-antagonist, physostigmine, neostigmine, sedative-hypnotics, chlorpromazine, verapamil, hypothermia, hyponatremia, hypoosmolality, pregnancy, Δ-9-tetrahydrocannabinol; MAC increased by MAO inhibitors, ephedrine, levodopa, chronic ethanol abuse, hypernatremia, hyperthermia, acute cocaine and acute amphetamine ingestion.

Guidelines/Precautions

1. Patients with stenotic lesions of the aortic or mitral valves poorly tolerate changes in blood pressure and systemic vascular resistance.
2. The MAC is highest in the first 6 months of life and is slightly lower in neonates. Beyond adolescence, anesthetic requirements decrease with age so that an 80-year-old patient should require only three fourths the alveolar concentration for anesthesia required for a young adult.
3. Produces dose-related depression of uterine contractility and tone, which can contribute to perioperative blood loss.
4. Crosses the placental barrier; the degree of fetal and neonatal depression (hypotension, hypoxia, acidosis) is directly proportional to the depth and duration of maternal anesthesia.
5. Changes in mental function may persist beyond the period of anesthetic administration and the immediate postoperative period. There may be altered psychomotor performance and driving skills.
6. Contraindicated in patients with known or suspected genetic susceptibility to malignant hyperthermia.
7. Abrupt onset of malignant hyperthermia may be triggered by sevoflurane. Early premonitory signs include muscle rigidity, especially jaw muscles, tachycardia and tachypnea unrespon-

sive to increased depth of anesthesia, evidence of increased oxygen consumption and carbon dioxide production (change in color and increased temperature of the carbon dioxide absorber), rising body temperature and metabolic acidosis.

Principal Adverse Reactions

Cardiovascular: Hypotension, arrhythmias.
Pulmonary: Respiratory depression, apnea.
CNS: Dizziness, euphoria, increased cerebral blood flow and intracranial pressure.
GI/Hepatic: Nausea, vomiting, ileus.
GU: Renal dysfunction.
Metabolic: Malignant hyperthermia.

BIBLIOGRAPHY

Attia RR et al, editors: *Practical anesthetic pharmacology,* New York, 1987, Appleton-Century-Crofts.

Barash P et al, editors: *Clinical anesthesia,* Philadelphia, 1989, JB Lippincott.

Berk JL et al, editors: *Handbook of critical care,* Boston, 1990, Little Brown.

Berry FA et al, editors: *Anesthetic management of difficult and routine pediatric patients,* New York, 1990, Churchill Livingstone.

Drug facts and comparisons, Philadelphia, 1992, JB Lippincott.

American Hospital Formulary Service: *Drug information.* Bethesda, Md, 1992, American Society of Hospital Pharmacists.

Estefanous FG, editor: *Opioids in anesthesia,* Boston, 1991, Butterworth.

Gilman AG et al, editors: *Goodman and Gilman's the pharmacological basis of therapeutics,* 1990, New York, Macmillan.

Goth A et al, editors: *Medical pharmacology,* St Louis, 1984, Mosby-Year Book.

Hensley FA et al, editors: *The practice of cardiac anesthesia,* Boston, 1990, Little Brown.

Kaplan JA, editor: *Cardiac anesthesia,* Philadelphia, 1987, WB Saunders.

Miller RD et al, editors: *Anesthesia,* New York, 1990, Churchill Livingstone.

Opie LH et al, editors: *Drugs for the heart,* Philadelphia, 1987, WB Saunders.

Physician's desk reference, Oradell, NJ, 1992, Medical Economics.

Ryan JF et al, editors: *A practice of anesthesia for infants and children,* Philadelphia, 1986, WB Saunders.

Scott DB et al, editors: *Techniques of regional anesthesia,* Norwalk, Conn, 1989, Appleton & Lange.

Shnider SM et al, editors: *Anesthesia for obstetrics,* Baltimore, 1987, Williams & Wilkins.

Stoelting RK, editor: *Pharmacology and physiology in anesthetic practice,* Philadelphia, 1991, JB Lippincott.

Wood M, editor: *Drugs and anesthesia,* Baltimore, 1990, Williams & Wilkins.

Appendix A

MALIGNANT HYPERTHERMIA PROTOCOL

1. Discontinue all inhalation anesthetics.
2. Hyperventilate with 100% oxygen (15–20 L/min).
3. Change the anesthesia circuit and soda lime cannister.
4. If possible, get another machine and use a nonrebreathing circuit.
5. Establish lines: a wide-bore cannula for CVP, arterial line (if not already in place), Foley catheter, nasogastric tube. Replace all potassium-containing IV fluids (e.g., lactated Ringer's) with normal saline.
6. Administer dantrolene (initial IV dose 2.5 mg/kg; titrate further doses as required; maximum dose 10 mg/kg).
   - Dantrolene must be mixed with sterile, distilled water.
   - A 70-kg patient will require 9–10 vials (20 mg in each vial) immediately.
   - Remember each vial of dantrolene also contains mannitol, 3 g.
7. Start cooling techniques for rapidly increasing temperatures and for those above 40° C:
   - Surface cooling with the patient on a cooling blanket and packed with ice.
   - Gastric, rectal, or peritoneal lavage with iced saline.
   - Iced IV fluids.
   - Pump bypass with a heat exchanger.
   Cooling should be stopped when the patient's temperature falls below 38° C to prevent inadvertent hypothermia.
8. Treat acidosis with sodium bicarbonate (1–2 mEq/kg initial dose, and titrate as necessary).
9. Treat hyperkalemia with sodium bicarbonate, insulin (0.15 unit/kg), and 20% dextrose (500 mg/kg).
10. Treat arrhythmias with procainamide slow IV, 3 mg/kg; maximum, 15 mg/kg.
11. Maintain urine output with mannitol or furosemide.
12. Provide energy substrate with 20% to 50% dextrose with insulin.
13. Provide cardiorespiratory support.
14. Monitor urine output, serum potassium and calcium levels, and arterial blood gases and perform clotting studies.
15. Monitor patient in the ICU for at least 24 hours.

16. Follow creatine phosphokinase, calcium, and potassium levels until they return to normal
17. Observe patient for disseminated intravascular coagulation.
18. Convert to oral dantrolene when extubated and stable (PO, 4–8 mg/kg/day in 3 divided doses for up to 3 days after the crisis).
19. Counsel patient.

**MALIGNANT HYPERTHERMIA HOTLINE
(209) 634–4917
ASK FOR INDEX ZERO MALIGNANT HYPERTHERMIA CONSULTANT LIST**

Appendix B

CARDIOPULMONARY RESUSCITATION
ALGORITHMS

TABLE B–1.

Ventricular Fibrillation (and Pulseless Ventricular Tachycardia)*†

```
    Witnessed arrest                    Unwitnessed arrest
          ↓                                    ↓
Check pulse—If no pulse            Check pulse—If no pulse
          ↓
   Precordial thump
          ↓
Check pulse—If no pulse
                                           ↓
              CPR until a defibrillator is available
                             ↓
            Check monitor for rhythm—If VF or VT
                             ↓
                  Defibrillate, 200 joules‡
                             ↓
               Defibrillate, 200–300 joules‡
                             ↓
            Defibrillate with up to 360 joules‡
                             ↓
                     CPR If no pulse
                             ↓
                 Establish IV access
                             ↓
     Epinephrine, 1:10,000, 0.5–1.0 mg IV push§
                             ↓
                 Intubate if possible.¶
                             ↓
            Defibrillate with up to 360 joules‡
                             ↓
               Lidocaine, 1 mg/kg IV push
                             ↓
            Defibrillate with up to 360 joules‡
                             ↓
               Bretylium, 5 mg/kg IV push‖
                             ↓
                (Consider bicarbonate)**
                             ↓
```

(Continued.)

TABLE B–1   (cont.).

Defibrillate with up to 360 joules‡

↓

Bretylium, 10 mg/kg IV push‖

↓

Defibrillate with up to 360 joules‡

↓

Repeat lidocaine or bretylium

↓

Defibrillate with up to 360 joules‡

*From: Guidelines for cardiopulmonary resuscitation and emergency cardiac care. *JAMA* 1986; 255:2948. Used with permission. This sequence was developed to assist in teaching how to treat a broad range of patients with ventricular fibrillation (VF) or pulseless ventricular tachycardia (VT). Some patients may require care not specified herein. This algorithm should not be construed as prohibiting such flexibility. Flow of algorithm presumes that VF is continuing. CPR indicates cardiopulmonary resuscitation.

†Pulseless VT should be treated identically to VF.

‡Check pulse and rhythm after each shock. If VF recurs after transiently converting (rather than persists without ever converting), use whatever energy level has previously been successful for defibrillation.

§Epinephrine should be repeated every five minutes.

¶Intubation is preferable. If it can be accompanied simultaneously with other techniques, then the earlier the better. However, defibrillation and epinephrine are more important initially if the patient can be ventilated without intubation.

‖Some may prefer repeated doses of lidocaine, which may be given in 0.5-mg/kg boluses every eight minutes to a total dose of 3 mg/kg.

**Value of sodium bicarbonate is questionable during cardiac arrest, and it is not recommended for routine cardiac arrest sequence. Consideration of its use in a dose of 1 mEq/kg is appropriate at this point. Half of original dose may be repeated every ten minutes if it is used.

TABLE B-2.

Asystole (Cardiac Standstill)*

If rhythm is unclear and possibly ventricular
fibrillation, defibrillate as for VF. If asystole is present†

↓

Continue CPR

↓

Establish IV access

↓

Epinephrine, 1:10,000, 0.5–1.0 mg IV push‡

↓

Intubate when possible§

↓

Atropine, 1.0 mg IV push (repeated in 5 min)

↓

(Consider bicarbonate)¶

↓

Consider pacing

*From: Guidelines for cardiopulmonary resuscitation and emergency cardiac care. *JAMA* 1986; 255:2948. Used with permission. This sequence was developed to assist in teaching how to treat a broad range of patients with asystole. Some patients may require care not specified herein. This algorithm should not be construed to prohibit such flexibility. Flow of algorithm presumes asystole is continuing. VF indicates ventricular fibrillation; IV, intravenous.

†Asystole should be confirmed in two leads.

‡Epinephrine should be repeated every five minutes.

§Intubation is preferable; if it can be accomplished simultaneously with other techniques, then the earlier the better. However, cardiopulmonary resuscitation (CPR) and use of epinephrine are more important initially if patient can be ventilated without intubation. (Endotracheal epinephrine may be used.)

¶Value of sodium bicarbonate is questionable during cardiac arrest, and it is not recommended for the routine cardiac arrest sequence. Consideration of its use in a dose of 1 mEq/kg is appropriate at this point. Half of original dose may be repeated every ten minutes if it is used.

TABLE B–3.

Electromechanical Dissociation*

Continue CPR

↓

Establish IV access

↓

Epinephrine, 1:10,000, 0.5–1.0 mg IV push†

↓

Intubate when possible‡

↓

(Consider bicarbonate)§

↓

Consider hypovolemia,
cardiac tamponade,
Tension pneumothorax,
Hypoxemia,
acidosis,
pulmonary embolism

*From: Guidelines for cardiopulmonary resuscitation and emergency cardiac care. *JAMA* 1986; 255:2948. Used with permission. This sequence was developed to assist in teaching how to treat a broad range of patients with electromechanical dissociation. Some patients may require care not specified herein. This algorithm should not be construed to prohibit such flexibility. Flow of algorithm presumes that electromechanical dissociation is continuing. CPR indicates cardiopulmonary resuscitation; IV, intravenous.

†Epinephrine should be repeated every five minutes.

‡Intubation is preferable. If it can be accomplished simultaneously with other techniques, then the earlier the better. However, epinephrine is more important initially if the patient can be ventilated without intubation.

§Value of sodium bicarbonate is questionable during cardiac arrest, and it is not recommended for routine cardiac arrest sequence. Consideration of its use in a dose of 1 mEq/kg is appropriate at this point. Half of original dose may be repeated every ten minutes if it is used.

TABLE B-4.

Sustainable Ventricular Tachycardia (VT)*

```
No pulse                        Pulse present
   ↓                                 |
Treat as VF         ┌────────────────┴────────────────┐
                  Stable†                          Unstable‡
                     ↓                                 ↓
                    O₂                                O₂
                     ↓                                 ↓
                 IV access                         IV access
                     ↓                                 ↓
            Lidocaine, 1 mg/kg                (Consider sedation)§
                     ↓                                 ↓
        Lidocaine, 0.5 mg/kg every 8 min      Cardiovert 50 joules¶,‖
           until VT resolves, or                     ↓
              up to 3 mg/kg                   Cardiovert 100 joules¶
                     ↓                                 ↓
         Procainamide, 20 mg/min             Cardiovert 200 joules¶
             until VT resolves,                      ↓
            or up to 1,000 mg               Cardiovert with up to
                     ↓                            360 joules¶
            Cardiovert as in                        ↓
            unstable patients'            If recurrent, add lidocaine
                                          and cardiovert again starting
                                              at energy level
                                          previously successful; then
                                          procainamide or bretylium**
```

*From: Guidelines for cardiopulmonary resuscitation and emergency cardiac care. *JAMA* 1986; 255:2948. Used with permission. This sequence was developed to assist in teaching how to treat a broad range of patients with sustained VT. Some patients may require care not specified herein. This algorithm should not be construed as prohibiting such flexibility. Flow of algorithm presumes that VT is continuing. VF indicates ventricular fibrillation.

†If patient becomes unstable (see next footnote for definition) at any time, move to "Unstable" arm of algorithm.

‡Unstable indicates symptoms (e.g., chest pain or dyspnea), hypotension (systolic blood pressure <90 mm Hg), congestive heart failure, ischemia, or infarction.

§Sedation should be considered for all patients, including those defined in footnote above as unstable, except those who are hemodynamically unstable (e.g., hypotensive, in pulmonary edema, or unconscious).

¶If hypotension, pulmonary edema, or unconsciousness is present, unsynchronized cardioversion should be done to avoid delay associated with synchronization.

‖In the absence of hypotension, pulmonary edema, or unconsciousness, a precordial thump may be employed prior to cardioversion.

**Once VT has resolved, begin intravenous (IV) infusion of antiarrhythmic agent that has aided resolution of VT. If hypotension, pulmonary edema, or unconsciousness is present, use lidocaine if cardioversion alone is unsuccessful, followed by bretylium. In all other patients, recommended order of therapy is lidocaine, procainamide, and then bretylium.

TABLE B-5.

Bradycardia*

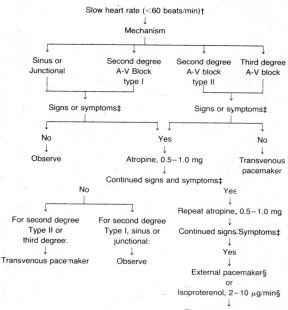

*From: Guidelines for cardiopulmonary resuscitation and emergency cardiac care. *JAMA* 1986; 255:2948. Used with permission. This sequence was developed to assist in teaching how to treat a broad range of patients with bradycardia. Some patients may require care not specified herein. This algorithm should not be construed to prohibit such flexibility. AV indicates atrioventricular.

†A solitary chest thump or cough may stimulate cardiac electrical activity and result in improved cardiac output and may be used at this point

‡Hypotension (blood pressure <90 mm Hg), premature ventricular contractions, altered mental status or symptoms (e.g., chest pain or dyspnea), ischemia, or infarction.

†Temporizing therapy.

TABLE B-6.

Ventricular Ectopy: Acute Suppressive Therapy*

Assess for need for
acute suppressive therapy

↓

→ Rule out treatable cause
→ Consider serum potassium
→ Consider digitalis level
→ Consider bradycardia
→ Consider drugs

Lidocaine, 1 mg/kg

↓

If not suppressed
repeat lidocaine, 0.5 mg/kg every 2-5 min,
until no ectopy, or up to 3 mg/kg given

↓

If not suppressed,
procainamide, 20 mg/min,
until no ectopy, or up to 1,000 mg given

↓

If not suppressed,
and not contraindicated,
bretylium, 5-10 mg/kg over 8-10 min

↓

If not suppressed,
consider overdrive pacing

Once ectopy resolved, maintain as follows:
  After lidocaine, 1 mg/kg . . . lidocaine drip, 2 mg/min
  after lidocaine, 1-2 mg/kg . . . lidocaine drip, 3 mg/min
  After lidocaine, 2-3 mg/kg . . . lidocaine drip, 4 mg/min
  After procainamide . . . procainamide drip, 1-4 mg/min (check blood level)
  After bretylium . . . bretylium drip, 2 mg/min

*From: Guidelines for cardiopulmonary resuscitation and emergency cardiac
care. *JAMA* 1986; 255:2948. Used with permission. This sequence was developed to assist in teaching how to treat a broad range of patients with ventricular
ectopy. Some patients may require therapy not specified herein. This algorithm
should not be construed as prohibiting such flexibility.

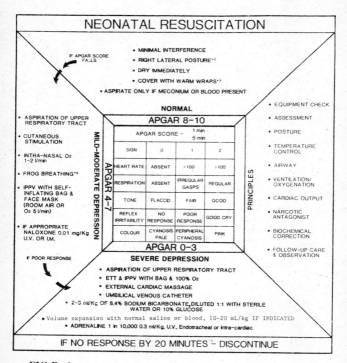

NEONATAL RESUSCITATION

IF APGAR SCORE FALLS
- MINIMAL INTERFERENCE
- RIGHT LATERAL POSTURE*[2]
- DRY IMMEDIATELY
- COVER WITH WARM WRAPS*[3]
- ASPIRATE ONLY IF MECONIUM OR BLOOD PRESENT

NORMAL
APGAR 8–10

- ASPIRATION OF UPPER RESPIRATORY TRACT
- CUTANEOUS STIMULATION
- INTRA-NASAL O_2 1–2 l/min
- FROG BREATHING*[4]
- IPPV WITH SELF-INFLATING BAG & FACE MASK (ROOM AIR OR O_2 5 l/min)
- IF APPROPRIATE NALOXONE 0.01 mg/Kg U.V. OR I.M.

MILD–MODERATE DEPRESSION
APGAR 4–7

APGAR SCORE –	1 min		
	5 min		
SIGN	0	1	2
HEART RATE	ABSENT	<100	>100
RESPIRATION	ABSENT	IRREGULAR GASPS	REGULAR
TONE	FLACCID	FAIR	GOOD
REFLEX IRRITABILITY	NO RESPONSE	POOR RESPONSE	GOOD CRY
COLOUR	CYANOSIS PALE	PERIPHERAL CYANOSIS	PINK

APGAR 0–3
SEVERE DEPRESSION

IF POOR RESPONSE
- ASPIRATION OF UPPER RESPIRATORY TRACT
- ETT & IPPV WITH BAG & 100% O_2
- EXTERNAL CARDIAC MASSAGE
- UMBILICAL VENOUS CATHETER
- 2–3 ml/Kg OF 8.4% SODIUM BICARBONATE, DILUTED 1:1 WITH STERILE WATER OR 10% GLUCOSE
- Volume expansion with normal saline or blood, 10–20 mL/kg IF INDICATED
- ADRENALINE 1 in 10,000 0.3 ml/Kg, U.V, Endotracheal or intra-cardiac

PRINCIPLES
- EQUIPMENT CHECK
- ASSESSMENT
- POSTURE
- TEMPERATURE CONTROL
- AIRWAY
- VENTILATION/ OXYGENATION
- CARDIAC OUTPUT
- NARCOTIC ANTAGONIST
- BIOCHEMICAL CORRECTION
- FOLLOW-UP CARE & OBSERVATION

IF NO RESPONSE BY 20 MINUTES – DISCONTINUE

FIG B–1.

The Melbourne chart. Notes: **1,** use of the chart: this chart uses the Apgar score to guide the user to the appropriate level of resuscitation. Normal infants (Apgar scores 8–10 at 1 minute) are pink. Mild to moderately depressed infants (Apgar score at 1 minute 4–7) approximately correspond to those with primary apnea, with intact circulation, and are blue. Severely depressed infants (Apgar score 0–3 at 1 minute) approximately correspond to those with secondary apnea, with depressed circulation, and are gray or white. **2,** posture: for normal and mildly depressed infants, the right lateral posture creates a spontaneously clear airway and minimizes the need for suction. The supine posture is indicated once IPPV with bag and mask is required. **3,** wraps: the wrap used to "catch" the infant should be used for the initial drying, then immediately discarded and replaced with a warm wrap. **4,** frog breathing: with intranasal oxygen at 1–2 L/min, the nares and mouth are simultaneously closed for 1–2 sec, thus forcing O_2 into the upper airway and stimulating Head's reflex. This causes a gasp in the majority of infants, sometimes followed by brief apnea. The process may be repeated every few seconds until respiration is established. Failure to elicit a gasp within 30 seconds should lead to bag and mask ventilation. **5,** response: "no response" is defined as no assessable improvement in heart rate, perfusion, color, or spontaneous respiration. In practice if there has been no gasp by 20 min—provided there is no respiratory depression from narcotics or hyperventilation—then the outlook is universally bad, either from death or severe morbidity, and discontinuation of resuscitative efforts should be considered. (From Roy RN, Betheras FR: *Anaesth Intensive Care* 1990; 18:350. Used by permission.)

Appendix C

INCOMPATIBILITY TABLE

Physical and Chemical Compatibility for Mixing and Infusing Medications*†

	Aminophylline	Ampicillin	Atropine sulfate	Bretylium	Calcium chloride	Calcium gluconate	Cefazolin	Cimetidine	Diazepam	Diazoxide	Digoxin	Dobutamine	Dopamine	Epinephrine HCl	Furosemide	Gentamicin	Heparin	Hydralazine	Insulin, regular	Isoproterenol
Verapamil	P	P	P	P	P	P	P	P	N	N	Z	N	–	P	P	P	P	P	S	P
Tobramy.	N	Z	N	Z	Z	–	–	Z	N	Z	Z	N	Z	Z	Z	Z	Z	–	Z	Z
Streptokinase	N	Z	Z	Z	N	Z	N	Z	N	Z	Z	Z	Z	Z	Z	Z	Z	Z	N	Z
Sodium bicarbonate	B	Z	–	C	–	–	Z	N	P	Z	Z	Z	N	–	–	Z	Z	P	Z	–
Quinidine	N	Z	Z	Z	P	Z	Z	Z	P	–	Z	Z	Z	Z	Z	–	Z	–	Z	Z
Propranolol	N	Z	Z	Z	P	Z	Z	Z	P	–	Z	Z	Z	Z	Z	–	Z	–	Z	Z
Procainamide	N	Z	P	–	Z	Z	Z	Z	Z	N	Z	P	Z	Z	Z	Z	P	Z	Z	N
Potassium chloride	P	P	P	P	P	P	S	D	Z	Z	Y	–	P	P	P	P	Z	P	Y	Z
Phytonadione	Z	–	Z	Z	Z	P	Z	P	Z	Z	Z	–	P	–	Z	Z	P	Z	Z	Z
Phenytoin	Z	Z	Z	Z	P	Z	N	Z	Z	Z	Z	Z	Z	Z	Z	Z	Z	Z	Z	Z
Norepinephrine	–	P	Z	Z	P	Z	N	D	Z	Z	Z	Z	P	H	P	Z	P	Z	P	Z
Nitroprusside	Z	Z	Z	Z	Z	Z	Z	Z	Z	Z	Z	Z	Z	Z	Z	Z	Z	Z	Z	Z
Nitroglycerin	G	Z	N	Z	G	Z	Z	Z	Z	Z	Z	Z	Z	G	Z	N	Z	G	Z	N
Netilmicin	N	Z	Z	Z	N	Z	N	P	Z	Z	Z	Z	Z	Z	Z	Z	Z	Z	Z	Z
Morphine sulfate	–	Z	P	Z	N	–	Z	Z	Z	Z	Z	Z	Z	Z	N	H	–	Z	Z	N
Lidocaine	P	P	N	C	P	D	–	D	Z	N	P	P	P	–	Z	P	P	P	L	–
Isoproterenol	P	–	N	–	P	P	N	P	Z	N	P	–	Z	N	P	P	P	N	–	–
Insulin, regular	–	Z	N	P	Z	Z	Z	A	Z	Z	–	–	Z	Z	N	Z	Z	Z	–	N
Hydralazine	–	–	Z	Z	N	Z	Z	Z	–	–	H	S	–	–	Z	N	–	P	–	P
Heparin	P	H	P	Z	N	Z	P	S	P	Z	Z	Z	D	S	P	A	–	D	P	P
Gentamicin	P	–	Z	N	M	Z	Z	–	Z	Z	Z	B	Z	A	Z	–	–	Z	Z	Z
Furosemide	B	Z	D	N	Z	Z	Z	Z	P	Z	Z	–	N	–	–	Z	P	N	–	Z
Epinephrine HCl	–	–	D	–	Z	Z	–	N	P	Z	Z	Z	D	–	–	P	D	P	–	Z
Dopamine	P	–	Z	C	D	D	P	Z	P	Z	Z	S	–	–	P	A	Z	P	Z	P
Dobutamine	B	Z	P	–	–	–	Z	P	Z	Z	Z	–	S	D	–	B	D	S	–	P
Digoxin	P	Z	Z	D	P	Z	Z	M	Z	Z	–	Z	Z	Z	Z	Z	H	–	Z	N
Diazoxide	Z	Z	Z	Z	Z	Z	Z	Z	Z	–	Z	Z	Z	Z	Z	Z	Z	–	Z	N
Diazepam	Z	Z	Z	Z	Z	Z	Z	–	–	Z	Z	Z	–	Z	Z	Z	Z	Z	Z	N
Cimetidine	–	A	P	Z	Z	Z	P	–	Z	Z	M	P	P	P	P	P	P	P	A	P
Cefazolin	S	S	Z	Z	Z	Z	–	–	P	Z	Z	Z	Z	Z	Z	–	–	S	Z	Z
Calcium gluconate	P	–	Z	D	Z	Z	–	–	Z	Z	Z	Z	–	P	–	Z	Z	P	Z	P
Calcium chloride	Z	Z	Z	C	–	–	Z	Z	Z	Z	P	–	D	–	Z	Z	Z	Z	Z	N
Bretylium	D	Z	Z	–	C	D	Z	Z	Z	Z	D	–	C	Z	Z	M	Z	Z	P	–
Atropine sulfate	Z	Z	–	–	Z	Z	N	Z	Z	Z	D	–	Z	D	Z	H	P	Z	Z	Z
Ampicillin	P	–	Z	Z	N	–	S	S	A	Z	Z	Z	Z	Z	N	–	Z	H	Z	P
Aminophylline	–	P	Z	D	Z	N	P	–	S	S	–	N	Z	N	B	P	–	P	–	–

Lidocaine	P	P	N	C	P	D	I	D	B	B	P	I	N	P	I	N	N	P	P	N	N	D	N	N	P
Morphine sulfate	I	N	P	I		N	N	N	N	N	N	N	N	N	N	N	N	P	N	N	I	N	N	
Netilmicin	N	N	P	G	N	N	N	G	N	N	N	P	N	B	B	B	B	N	N	P	B	N		
Nitroglycerin	G	N	N	N	N	N	G	N	N	P	N	N	N	N	N	B	N	N	N	N	N			
Nitroprusside	N	N	N	N	N	N	P	N	N	N	N	N	N	N	N	N	N	N	P					
Norepinephrine	I	P	N	P	N	D	H	P	P	N	I	N	N	N	N	N	I	N						
Phenytoin	N	N	N	N	N	N	N	N	N	N	N	N	N	N	N	N	N							
Phytonadione	N	I	N	N	P	I	P	I	P	N	P	P	N	P	N	N	N							
Potassium chloride	P	P	P	P	P	N	P	Y	N	N	N	P	P	N	N									
Procainamide	N	N	P	I	P	N	N	N	N	P	N	N	N	N										
Propranolol	N	N	N	N	N	N	N	N	N	N	N	N	N											
Quinidine	N	N	P	N	I		N	N		I	N	N	P											
Sodium bicarbonate	B	N		C	I		D	I	N	N	N	N												
Streptokinase	N	N	N	I		N	N	N	N	N	N													
Tobramycin	N	N	N	I		I	N	N	N	P	N													
Verapamil	P	P	P	P	P	P	P	I	P	P	P	P	S	P	P									

*From Zeller FP, Anders R: *Drug Intell Clin Pharm* 1986; 20:349–352. Used with permission.
†C = physically and chemically compatible; P = physically compatible; D = physically compatible only in D₅W; S = physically compatible only in 0.9% NaCl; G = physically compatible only in a glass bottle; H = physically compatible for 4–8 hr; B = physically compatible for 4–8 hr only in D₅W; Y = physically compatible through Y-site for at least 6 hr; L = regular insulin compatible with preservative-free lidocaine solution; M = manufacturer claims medication should not be mixed with other medications but some compatibility data are available; I = incompatible; N = information on compatibility is not available.

Appendix D

INFUSION TABLES

Sota Omoigui M.D.
Didaciane Gatete, R.N.

Epidural Alfentanil 1500 µg in 150
mL (10 µg/ml)*

µg/hr	ml/hr
100	10
110	11
120	12
130	13
140	14
150	15
160	16
170	17
180	18
190	19
200	20
210	21
220	22
230	23
240	24
250	25

*Data from *The Criticare Drug Dose and
Infusion Calculator Software.* Mt Vernon, Ill, Med-Pharm Information Systems, 1991.

Intravenous Alfentanil, 10 mg in 250 mL (40 µg/mL)†

Dose, µg/kg/min	Patient's Weight (lb/kg)														
	66/30	77/35	88/40	99/45	110/50	121/55	132/60	143/65	154/70	165/75	176/80	187/85	198/90	209/95	220/100
	Infusion Rate, ml/hr														
0.1	5	5	6	7	8	8	9	10	11	11	12	13	14	14	15
0.2	9	11	12	14	15	17	18	20	21	23	24	26	27	29	30
0.3	14	16	18	20	23	25	27	29	32	34	36	38	41	43	45
0.4	18	21	24	27	30	33	36	39	42	45	48	51	54	57	60
0.5	23	26	30	34	38	41	45	49	53	56	60	64	68	71	75
0.6	27	32	36	41	45	50	54	59	63	68	72	77	81	86	90
0.7	32	37	42	47	53	58	63	68	74	78	84	89	95	100	105
0.8	36	42	48	54	60	66	72	78	84	90	96	102	108	114	120
0.9	41	47	54	61	68	74	81	88	95	101	108	115	122	128	135
1.0	45	53	60	68	75	83	90	98	105	113	120	128	135	143	150
2.0	90	105	120	135	150	165	180	195	210	225	240	255	270	285	300
3.0	135	158	180	202	225	248	270	293	315	338	360	383	405	428	450

*Data from *The Criticare Drug Dose and Infusion Calculator Software*, Mt Vernon, III; Med-Pharm Information Systems, 1991.
†Infusion rate is found at intersection of "Dose" and Patient's Weight columns.

Aminocaproic Acid, 15 g in 500
mL (30 mg/mL)*

g/hr	mL/hr
0.5	17
0.6	20
0.7	23
0.8	27
0.9	30
1	33
1.1	37
1.2	40
1.25	42

*Data from *The Criticare Drug Dose and Infusion Calculator Software.* Mt Vernon, Ill, Med-Pharm Information Systems, 1991.

Aminophylline, 500 mg in 500 mL (1 mg/mL)*†

Dose, mg/kg/hr	Patient's Weight (lb/kg)														
	66/30	77/35	88/40	99/45	110/50	121/55	132/60	143/65	154/70	165/75	176/80	187/85	198/90	209/95	220/100
	Infusion Rate, mL/hr														
0.1	3	4	4	5	5	6	6	6	7	8	8	9	9	10	10
0.2	6	7	8	9	10	11	12	13	14	15	16	17	18	19	20
0.3	9	11	12	14	15	17	18	20	21	23	24	26	27	29	30
0.4	12	14	16	18	20	22	24	26	28	30	32	34	36	38	40
0.5	15	18	20	23	25	28	30	33	35	38	40	43	45	48	50
0.6	18	21	24	27	30	33	36	39	42	45	48	51	54	57	60
0.7	21	25	28	32	35	39	42	46	49	53	56	60	63	67	70
0.8	24	28	32	36	40	44	48	52	56	60	64	68	72	76	80
0.9	27	32	36	41	45	50	54	59	63	68	72	77	81	86	90
1.0	30	35	40	45	50	55	60	65	70	75	80	85	90	95	100

*Data from The Criticare Drug Dose and Infusion Calculator Software. Mt Vernon, Ill, Med-Pharm Information Systems, 1991.
†Infusion rate is found at intersection of "Dose" and Patient's Weight columns.

Amrinone, 500 mg in 500 mL (1 mg/mL)*†

Infusion Rate, mL/hr

Dose, µg/kg/min	Patient's Weight (lb/kg)														
	66/30	77/35	88/40	99/45	110/50	121/55	132/60	143/65	154/70	165/75	176/80	187/85	198/90	209/95	220/100
1	2	2	2	3	3	3	4	4	4	5	5	5	5	6	6
2	4	4	5	5	6	7	7	8	8	9	10	10	11	11	12
3	5	6	7	8	9	10	11	12	13	14	14	15	16	17	18
4	7	8	10	11	12	13	14	16	17	18	19	20	22	23	24
5	9	11	12	14	15	17	18	20	21	23	24	26	27	29	30
6	11	13	14	16	18	20	22	23	25	27	29	31	32	34	36
7	13	15	17	19	21	23	25	27	29	32	34	36	38	40	42
8	14	17	19	22	24	26	29	31	34	36	38	41	43	46	48
9	16	19	22	24	27	30	32	35	38	41	43	46	49	51	54
10	18	21	24	27	30	33	36	39	42	45	48	51	54	57	60
11	20	23	26	30	33	36	40	43	46	50	53	56	59	63	66
12	22	25	29	32	36	40	43	47	50	54	58	61	65	68	72
13	23	27	31	35	39	43	47	51	55	59	62	66	70	74	78
14	25	29	34	38	42	46	50	55	59	63	67	71	76	80	84
15	27	32	36	41	45	50	54	59	63	68	72	77	81	86	90
16	29	34	38	43	48	53	58	62	67	72	77	82	87	91	96
17	31	36	41	46	51	56	61	66	71	77	82	87	92	97	102
18	32	38	43	49	54	59	65	70	76	81	86	92	97	103	108
19	34	40	46	51	57	63	68	74	80	86	91	97	103	108	114

*Data from The Criticare Drug Dose and Infusion Calculator Software. Mt Vernon, Ill, Med-Pharm Information Systems, 1991.
†Infusion rate is found at intersection of "Dose" and Patient's Weight columns.

Atracurium, 20 mg in 100 mL (0.2 mg/mL)*†

Patient's Weight $\left(\frac{lb}{kg}\right)$

Infusion Rate, mL/hr

Dose, µg/kg/min	66/30	77/35	88/40	99/45	110/50	121/55	132/60	143/65	154/70	165/75	176/80	187/85	198/90	209/95	220/100
1	9	11	12	14	15	17	18	20	21	22	24	26	27	29	30
2	18	21	24	27	30	33	36	39	42	45	48	51	54	57	60
3	27	32	36	41	45	50	54	59	63	68	72	77	81	86	90
4	36	42	48	54	60	66	72	78	84	90	96	102	108	114	120
5	45	53	60	68	75	83	90	98	105	113	120	128	135	143	150
6	54	63	72	81	90	99	108	117	126	135	144	153	162	171	180
7	63	74	84	95	105	116	126	137	147	158	168	179	189	200	210
8	72	84	96	108	120	132	144	156	168	180	192	204	216	228	240
9	81	95	108	122	135	149	162	176	189	203	216	230	243	257	270
10	90	105	120	135	150	165	180	195	210	225	240	255	270	285	300
11	99	116	132	149	165	182	198	215	231	248	264	281	297	314	330
12	108	126	144	162	180	198	216	234	252	270	288	306	324	342	360
13	117	137	156	176	195	215	234	254	273	293	312	332	351	371	390
14	126	147	168	189	210	231	252	273	294	315	336	357	378	399	420
15	135	158	180	203	225	248	270	293	315	338	360	383	405	428	450

*Data from The Criticare Drug Dose and Infusion Calculator Software. Mt Vernon, Ill, Med-Pharm Information Systems, 1991.
†Infusion rate is found at intersection of "Dose" and Patient's Weight columns.

Bretylium, 2 g in 500 mL
(4 mg/mL)*

mg/min	mL/hr
1	15
1.1	17
1.2	18
1.3	20
1.4	21
1.5	23
1.6	24
1.7	26
1.8	27
1.9	29
2	30

*Data from *The Criticare Drug Dose and Infusion Calculator Software.* Mt Vernon, Ill, Med-Pharm Information Systems, 1991.

Curare, 15 mg in 100 mL (0.15 mg/mL)*†

Dose, μg/kg/min	Patient's Weight (lb/kg)														
	66/30	77/35	88/40	99/45	110/50	121/55	132/60	143/65	154/70	165/75	176/80	187/85	198/90	209/95	220/100
	Infusion Rate, mL/hr														
1	12	14	16	18	20	22	24	26	28	30	32	34	36	38	40
2	24	28	32	36	40	44	48	52	56	60	64	68	72	76	80
3	36	42	48	54	60	66	72	78	84	90	96	102	108	114	120
4	48	56	64	72	80	88	96	104	112	120	128	136	144	152	160
5	60	70	80	90	100	110	120	130	140	150	160	170	180	190	200
6	72	84	96	108	120	132	144	156	168	180	192	204	216	228	240

*Data from The Criticare Drug Dose and Infusion Calculator Software. Mt Vernon, Ill, Med-Pharm Information Systems, 1991.
†Infusion rate is found at intersection of "Dose" and "Patient's Weight columns.

Dobutamine, 500 mg in 500 mL (1 mg/mL)*†

Dose, µg/kg/min	Patient's Weight lb/(kg) — Infusion Rate, mL/hr														
	66/30	77/35	88/40	99/45	110/50	121/55	132/60	143/65	154/70	165/75	176/80	187/85	198/90	209/95	220/100
2	4	4	5	5	6	7	7	8	8	9	10	10	11	11	12
4	7	8	10	11	12	13	14	16	17	18	19	20	22	23	24
6	11	13	14	16	18	20	22	23	25	27	29	31	32	34	36
8	14	17	19	22	24	26	29	31	34	36	38	41	43	46	48
10	18	21	24	27	30	33	36	39	42	45	48	51	54	57	60
12	22	25	29	32	36	40	43	47	50	54	58	61	65	68	72
14	25	29	34	38	42	46	50	55	59	63	67	71	76	80	84
16	29	34	38	43	48	53	58	62	67	72	77	82	86	91	96
18	32	38	43	49	54	59	65	70	76	81	86	92	97	103	108
20	36	42	48	54	60	66	72	78	84	90	96	102	108	114	120
22	40	46	53	59	66	73	80	86	92	99	106	112	119	125	132
24	43	50	58	65	72	79	86	94	101	108	115	122	130	137	144
26	47	55	62	70	78	86	94	101	109	117	125	133	140	148	156
28	50	59	67	76	84	92	101	109	118	126	134	143	151	160	168
30	54	63	72	81	90	99	108	117	126	135	144	153	162	171	180
32	58	67	77	86	96	106	115	125	134	144	154	163	173	182	192
34	61	71	82	92	102	112	122	133	143	153	163	173	184	194	204
36	65	76	86	97	108	119	130	140	151	162	173	184	194	205	216
38	68	80	91	103	114	125	137	148	160	171	182	194	205	217	228
40	72	84	96	108	120	132	144	156	168	180	192	204	216	228	240

*Data from *The Criticare Drug Dose and Infusion Calculator Software.* Mt Vernon, Ill, Med-Pharm Information Systems, 1991.
†Infusion rate is found at intersection of Dose and Patient's Weight columns.

Dopamine, 400 mg in 250 mL (1600 µg/mL)*†

Patient's Weight ($\frac{lb}{kg}$)

Infusion Rate, mL/hr

Dose, µg/kg/min	$\frac{66}{30}$	$\frac{77}{35}$	$\frac{88}{40}$	$\frac{99}{45}$	$\frac{110}{50}$	$\frac{121}{55}$	$\frac{132}{60}$	$\frac{143}{65}$	$\frac{154}{70}$	$\frac{165}{75}$	$\frac{176}{80}$	$\frac{187}{85}$	$\frac{198}{90}$	$\frac{209}{95}$	$\frac{220}{100}$
1	1	1	2	2	2	2	2	2	3	3	3	3	3	4	4
2	2	3	3	3	4	4	5	5	5	6	6	6	7	7	8
3	3	4	5	5	6	6	7	7	8	8	9	10	10	11	11
4	4	5	6	7	8	8	9	10	11	11	12	13	14	14	15
5	6	7	8	8	9	10	11	12	13	14	15	16	17	18	19
6	7	8	9	10	11	12	14	15	16	17	18	19	20	21	23
7	8	9	11	12	13	14	16	17	18	20	21	22	24	25	26
8	9	11	12	14	15	17	18	20	21	23	24	26	27	29	30
9	10	12	14	15	17	19	20	22	24	25	27	29	30	32	34
10	11	13	15	17	19	21	23	24	26	28	30	32	34	36	38
11	12	14	17	19	21	23	25	26	29	31	33	35	37	39	41
12	14	16	18	20	23	25	27	29	32	34	36	38	41	43	45
13	15	17	20	22	24	27	29	32	34	37	39	41	44	46	49
14	16	18	21	24	26	29	32	34	37	39	42	45	47	50	53
15	17	20	23	25	28	31	34	37	39	42	45	48	51	54	56
16	18	21	24	27	30	33	36	39	42	45	48	51	54	57	60
17	19	22	26	29	32	35	38	41	45	48	51	54	57	61	64
18	20	24	27	30	34	37	41	44	47	51	54	57	61	64	68
19	21	25	29	32	36	39	43	46	50	53	57	61	64	68	71
20	23	26	30	34	38	41	45	49	53	56	60	64	68	71	75

*Data from *The Criticare Drug Dose and Infusion Calculator Software.* Mt Vernon, Ill. Med-Pharm Information Systems, 1991.
†Infusion rate is found at intersection of "Dose" and Patient's Weight columns.

Doxapram, 250 mg in 250 mL
(1 mg/mL)*

mg/min	mL/hr
1	60
2	120
3	180
4	240
5	300

*Data from *The Criticare Drug Dose and Infusion Calculator Software.* Mt Vernon, Ill, Med-Pharm Information Systems, 1991.

Epinephrine, 3 mg in 250 mL
(12 µg/mL)*

µg/min	mL/hr
1	5
2	10
3	15
4	20
5	25
6	30
7	35
8	40
9	45
10	50
11	55
12	60
13	65
14	70
15	75
16	80
17	85
18	90
19	95
20	100

*Data from *The Criticare Drug Dose and Infusion Calculator Software.* Mt Vernon, Ill, Med-Pharm Information Systems, 1991.

Esmolol 5 g in 500 mL (10 mg/mL)†

Dose, µg/kg/min	Patient's Weight (lb) / (kg) — Infusion Rate, mL/hr														
	66 / 30	77 / 35	88 / 40	99 / 45	110 / 50	121 / 55	132 / 60	143 / 65	154 / 70	165 / 75	176 / 80	187 / 85	198 / 90	209 / 95	220 / 100
50	9	11	12	14	15	17	18	20	21	23	24	26	27	29	30
60	11	13	14	16	18	20	22	23	25	27	29	31	32	34	36
70	13	15	17	19	21	23	25	27	29	32	34	36	38	40	42
80	14	17	19	22	24	26	29	31	34	36	38	41	43	46	48
90	16	19	22	24	27	30	32	35	38	41	43	46	49	51	54
100	18	21	24	27	30	33	36	39	42	45	48	51	54	57	60
110	20	23	26	30	33	36	40	43	46	50	53	56	59	63	66
120	22	25	29	32	36	40	43	47	50	54	58	61	65	68	72
130	23	27	31	35	39	43	47	51	55	59	62	66	70	74	78
140	25	29	34	38	42	46	50	55	59	63	67	71	76	80	84
150	27	32	36	41	45	50	54	59	63	68	72	77	81	86	90
160	29	34	38	43	48	53	58	62	67	72	77	82	86	91	96
170	31	36	41	46	51	56	61	66	71	77	82	87	92	97	102
180	32	38	43	49	54	59	65	70	76	81	86	92	97	103	108
190	34	40	46	51	57	63	68	74	80	86	91	97	103	108	114
200	36	42	48	54	60	66	72	78	84	90	96	102	108	114	120
210	38	44	50	57	63	69	76	82	88	95	101	107	113	120	126
220	40	46	53	59	66	73	79	86	92	99	106	112	119	125	132
230	41	48	55	62	69	76	83	90	97	104	110	117	124	131	138
240	43	50	58	65	72	79	86	94	101	108	115	122	130	137	144
250	45	53	60	68	75	83	90	98	105	113	120	128	135	143	150

*Data from *The Criticare Drug Dose and Infusion Calculator Software,* Mt. Vernon, Ill; Med-Pharm Information Systems, 1991.
†Infusion rate is found at intersection of "Dose" and Patient's Weight columns.

Epidural Fentanyl, 500 µg in 100 mL Local Anesthetic (5 µg/mL)*

µg/hr	mL/hr
20	4
25	5
30	6
35	7
40	8
45	9
50	10
55	11
60	12

*Data from *The Criticare Drug Dose and Infusion Calculator Software.* Mt Vernon, Ill, Med-Pharm Information Systems, 1991.

Intravenous Fentanyl, 500 µg in 100 mL (5 µg/mL)*†

								Patient's Weight ($\frac{lb}{kg}$)							
Dose, µg/kg/min	$\frac{66}{30}$	$\frac{77}{35}$	$\frac{88}{40}$	$\frac{99}{45}$	$\frac{110}{50}$	$\frac{121}{55}$	$\frac{132}{60}$	$\frac{143}{65}$	$\frac{154}{70}$	$\frac{165}{75}$	$\frac{176}{80}$	$\frac{187}{85}$	$\frac{198}{90}$	$\frac{209}{95}$	$\frac{220}{100}$
								Infusion Rate, mL/hr							
0.05	18	21	24	27	30	33	36	39	42	45	48	51	54	57	60
0.06	22	25	29	32	36	40	43	47	50	54	58	61	65	68	72
0.07	25	29	34	38	42	46	50	55	59	63	67	71	76	80	84
0.08	29	34	38	43	48	53	58	62	67	72	77	82	86	91	96
0.09	32	39	43	49	54	59	65	70	76	81	86	92	97	103	108
0.1	36	42	48	54	60	66	72	78	84	90	96	102	108	114	120
0.11	40	46	53	59	66	73	79	86	92	99	106	112	119	125	132
0.12	43	50	58	65	72	79	86	94	101	108	115	122	130	137	144
0.13	47	55	62	70	78	86	94	101	109	117	125	133	140	148	156
0.14	50	59	67	76	84	92	101	109	118	126	134	143	151	160	168
0.15	54	63	72	81	90	99	108	117	126	135	144	153	162	171	180
0.16	58	67	77	86	96	106	115	125	134	144	154	163	173	182	192
0.17	61	71	82	92	102	112	122	133	143	153	163	173	184	194	204
0.18	65	76	86	97	108	119	130	140	151	162	173	184	194	205	216
0.19	68	80	91	103	114	125	137	148	160	171	182	194	205	217	228
0.2	72	84	96	108	120	132	144	156	168	180	192	204	216	228	240

*Data from *The Criticare Drug Dose and Infusion Calculator Software.* Mt Vernon, Ill, Med-Pharm Information Systems, 1991.
†Infusion rate is found at intersection of "Dose" and Patient's Weight columns.

Heparin, 25,000 Units in 250 mL
(100 Units/mL)*

Units/24 hr	Units/hr	mL/hr
19,200	800	8
21,600	900	9
24,000	1000	10
26,400	1100	11
28,800	1200	12
31,200	1300	13
33,600	1400	14
36,000	1500	15
38,400	1600	16
40,800	1700	17

*Data from *The Criticare Drug Dose and Infusion Calculator Software*. Mt Vernon, Ill, Med-Pharm Information Systems, 1991.

Epidural Hydromorphone, 5 mg
in 100 mL Local Anesthetic
(50 μg/mL)*

mg/hr	mL/hr
0.15	3
0.2	4
0.25	5
0.3	6

*Data from *The Criticare Drug Dose and Infusion Calculator Software*. Mt Vernon, Ill, Med-Pharm Information Systems, 1991.

Intravenous Hydromorphone, 5
mg in 100 mL (50 μg/mL)*

mg/hr	mL/hr
0.15	3
0.2	4
0.25	5
0.3	6

*Data from *The Criticare Drug Dose and Infusion Calculator Software.* Mt Vernon, Ill, Med-Pharm Information Systems, 1991.

Isoproterenol, 3 mg in 250 mL
(12 μg/mL)*

μg/min	mL/hr
0.5	3
1	5
2	10
3	15
4	20
5	25
6	30
7	35
8	40
9	45
10	50
11	55
12	60
13	65
14	70
15	75
16	80
17	85
18	90
19	95
20	100

*Data from *The Criticare Drug Dose and Infusion Calculator Software.* Mt Vernon, Ill, Med-Pharm Information Systems, 1991.

Ketamine, 250 mg in 250 mL (1 mg/mL)*†

Dose, µg/kg/min	Patient's Weight lb/kg														
	66/30	77/35	88/40	99/45	110/50	121/55	132/60	143/65	154/70	165/75	176/80	187/85	198/90	209/95	220/100
	Infusion Rate, mL/hr														
10	18	21	24	27	30	33	36	39	42	45	48	51	54	57	60
20	36	42	48	54	60	66	72	78	84	90	96	102	108	114	120
30	54	63	72	81	90	99	108	117	126	135	144	153	162	171	180
40	72	84	96	108	120	132	144	156	168	180	192	204	216	228	240
50	90	105	120	135	150	165	180	195	210	225	240	255	270	285	300
60	108	126	144	162	180	198	216	234	252	270	288	306	324	342	360
70	126	147	168	189	210	231	252	273	294	315	336	357	378	399	420
80	144	168	192	216	240	264	288	312	336	360	384	408	432	456	480

*Data from *The Criticare Drug Dose and Infusion Calculator Software*, Mt Vernon, Ill, Med-Pharm Information Systems, 1991.
†Infusion rate is found at intersection of "Dose" and Patient's Weight columns.

Labetalol, 200 mg in 200 mL
(1 mg/mL)*

mg/min	mL/hr
0.5	30
0.6	36
0.7	42
0.8	48
0.9	54
1	60
1.1	66
1.2	72
1.3	78
1.4	84
1.5	90
1.6	96
1.7	102
1.8	108
1.9	114
2	120

*Data from *The Criticare Drug Dose and Infusion Calculator Software.* Mt Vernon, Ill, Med-Pharm Information Systems, 1991.

Lidocaine, 2 g in 500 mL
(4 mg/mL)*

mg/min	mL/hr
0.5	8
1	15
1.5	23
2	30
2.5	38
3	45
3.5	53
4	60

*Data from *The Criticare Drug Dose and Infusion Calculator Software.* Mt Vernon, Ill, Med-Pharm Information Systems, 1991.

Magnesium Sulfate, 10 g in 1000 mL (10 mg/mL)*

g/hr	mL/hr
1	100
1.1	110
1.2	120
1.3	130
1.4	140
1.5	150
1.6	160
1.7	170
1.8	180
1.9	190
2	200

*Data from *The Criticare Drug Dose and Infusion Calculator Software.* Mt Vernon, Ill, Med-Pharm Information Systems, 1991.

Epidural Meperidine, 100 mg in 50 mL Local Anesthetic (2 mg/mL)*

mg/hr	mL/hr
10	5
12	6
14	7
16	8
18	9
20	10

*Data from *The Criticare Drug Dose and Infusion Calculator Software.* Mt Vernon, Ill, Med-Pharm Information Systems, 1991.

Mephentermine, 250 mg in 250 mL (1 mg/mL)

mg/min	mL/hr
0.25	15
0.5	30
1	60
1.5	90
2	120
2.5	150
3	180
3.5	210
4	240
4.5	270
5	300

*Data from *The Criticare Drug Dose and Infusion Calculator Software.* Mt Vernon, Ill, Med-Pharm Information Systems, 1991.

Methohexital, 500 mg in 50 mL (10 mg/mL)*†

Dose, µg/kg/min	Patient's Weight (lb/kg)														
	66/30	77/35	88/40	99/45	110/50	121/55	132/60	143/65	154/70	165/75	176/80	187/85	198/90	209/95	220/100
	Infusion Rate, mL/hr														
50	9	11	12	14	15	17	18	20	21	23	24	26	27	29	30
60	11	13	15	16	18	20	22	23	25	27	29	30	32	34	36
70	13	15	17	19	21	23	25	27	29	32	34	36	38	40	42
80	14	17	19	22	24	26	29	31	34	36	38	41	43	46	48
90	16	19	22	24	27	30	32	35	38	41	43	46	49	51	54
100	18	21	24	27	30	33	36	39	42	45	48	51	54	57	60
110	20	23	26	30	33	36	40	43	46	50	53	56	59	63	66
120	22	25	29	32	36	40	43	47	50	54	58	61	65	68	72
130	23	27	31	35	39	43	47	51	55	59	62	66	70	74	78
140	25	29	34	38	42	46	50	55	59	63	67	71	76	80	84
150	27	32	36	41	45	50	54	59	63	68	72	77	81	86	90

*Data from *The Criticare Drug Dose and Infusion Calculator Software*, Mt Vernon, Ill, Med-Pharm Information Systems, 1991.
†Infusion rate is found at intersection of *Dose* and *Patient's Weight* columns.

Midazolam, 15 mg in 250 mL (60 µg/mL)*†

Patient's Weight (lb/kg)

Infusion Rate, mL/hr

Dose, µg/kg/min	66/30	77/35	88/40	99/45	110/50	121/55	132/60	143/65	154/70	165/75	176/80	187/85	198/90	209/95	220/100
0.1	3	4	4	5	5	6	6	7	7	8	8	9	9	10	10
0.2	6	7	8	9	10	11	12	13	14	15	16	17	18	19	20
0.3	9	11	12	14	15	17	18	20	21	23	24	26	27	29	30
0.4	12	14	16	18	20	22	24	26	28	30	32	34	36	38	40
0.5	15	18	20	23	25	28	30	33	35	38	40	43	45	48	50
0.6	18	21	24	27	30	33	36	39	42	45	48	51	54	57	60
0.7	21	25	28	32	35	39	42	46	49	53	56	60	63	67	70
0.8	24	28	32	36	40	44	48	52	56	60	64	68	72	76	80
0.9	27	32	36	41	45	50	54	59	63	68	72	77	81	86	90
1	30	35	40	45	50	55	60	65	70	75	80	85	90	95	100
1.1	33	39	44	50	55	61	66	72	77	83	88	94	99	105	110
1.2	36	42	48	54	60	66	72	78	84	90	96	102	108	114	120
1.3	39	45	52	59	65	72	78	85	91	98	104	111	117	124	130
1.4	42	49	56	63	70	77	84	91	98	105	112	119	126	133	140
1.5	45	53	60	68	75	83	90	98	105	113	120	128	135	143	150

*Data from The Criticare Drug Dose and Infusion Calculator Software. Mt Vernon, Ill, Med-Pharm Information Systems, 1991.
†Infusion rate is found at intersection of 'Dose' and Patient's Weight columns.

Mivacurium Chloride, 25 mg in 50 mL (0.5 mg/mL)*†

Dose, μg/kg/min	Patient's Weight (lb / kg)														
	66/30	77/35	88/40	99/45	110/50	121/55	132/60	143/65	154/70	165/75	176/80	187/85	198/90	209/95	220/100
	Infusion Rate, mL/hr														
1	4	4	5	5	6	7	7	8	8	9	10	10	11	11	12
2	7	8	10	11	12	13	14	16	17	18	19	20	22	23	24
3	11	13	14	16	18	20	22	23	25	27	29	31	32	34	36
4	14	17	19	22	24	26	29	31	34	36	38	41	43	46	48
5	18	21	24	27	30	33	36	39	42	45	48	51	54	57	60
6	22	25	29	32	36	40	43	47	50	54	58	61	65	68	72
7	25	29	34	38	42	46	50	55	59	63	67	71	76	80	84
8	29	34	38	43	48	53	58	62	67	72	77	82	86	91	96
9	32	38	43	49	54	59	65	70	76	81	86	92	97	103	108
10	36	42	48	54	60	66	72	78	84	90	96	102	108	114	120
11	40	46	53	59	66	73	79	86	92	99	106	112	119	125	132
12	43	50	58	65	72	79	86	94	101	108	115	122	130	137	144
13	47	55	62	70	78	86	94	101	109	117	125	133	140	148	156
14	50	59	67	76	84	92	101	109	118	126	134	143	151	160	168
15	54	63	72	81	90	99	108	117	126	135	144	153	162	171	180

*Data from The Criticare Drug Dose and Infusion Calculator Software. Mt Vernon, Ill, Med-Pharm Information Systems, 1991.
†Infusion rate is found at intersection of "Dose" and Patient's Weight columns.

Oxytocin, 10 Units in 1000 mL (10 mU/mL)*

mU/min	mL/hr
2	12
4	24
6	36
8	48
10	60
12	72
14	84
16	96
18	108
20	120
22	132
24	144
26	156
28	168
30	180
32	192
34	204
36	216
38	228
40	240

*Data from *The Criticare Drug Dose and Infusion Calculator Software*. Mt Vernon, Ill, Med-Pharm Information Systems, 1991.

Epidural Morphine, 10 mg in 100 mL Local Anesthetic (0.1 mg/mL)*

mg/hr	mL/hr
0.1	1
0.2	2
0.3	3
0.4	4
0.5	5
0.6	6
0.7	7
0.8	8
0.9	9
1	10

*Data from *The Criticare Drug Dose and Infusion Calculator Software*. Mt Vernon, Ill, Med-Pharm Information Systems, 1991.

Nitroglycerin, 50 mg in 250 mL
(200 µg/mL)*

µg/min	mL/hr
10	3
20	6
30	9
40	12
50	15
60	18
70	21
80	24
90	27
100	30
110	33
120	36
130	39
140	42
150	45
160	48
170	51
180	54
190	57
200	60

*Data from *The Criticare Drug Dose and Infusion Calculator Software.* Mt Vernon, Ill, Med-Pharm Information Systems, 1991.

Norepinephrine, 8 mg in 500 mL (16 μg/mL)*

μg/min	mL/hr
1	4
2	8
3	11
4	15
5	19
6	23
7	26
8	30
9	34
10	38
11	41
12	45
13	49
14	53
15	56
16	60
17	64
18	68
19	71
20	75

*Data from *The Criticare Drug Dose and Infusion Calculator Software.* Mt Vernon, Ill, Med-Pharm Information Systems, 1991.

Phentolamine, 200 mg in 100 mL (2 mg/mL)*

mg/min	mL/hr
0.1	3
0.2	6
0.3	9
0.4	12
0.5	15
0.6	18
0.7	21
0.8	24
0.9	27
1	30

*Data from *The Criticare Drug Dose and Infusion Calculator Software.* Mt Vernon, Ill, Med-Pharm Information Systems, 1991.

Phenylephrine, 30 mg in 500 mL
(60 μg/mL)*

μg/min	mL/hr
10	10
20	20
30	30
40	40
50	50
60	60
70	70
80	80
90	90
100	100
110	110
120	120
130	130
140	140
150	150
160	160
170	170
180	180
190	190
200	200

*Data from *The Criticare Drug Dose and Infusion Calculator Software.* Mt Vernon, Ill, Med-Pharm Information Systems, 1991.

Procainamide, 2 g in 500 mL
(4 mg/mL)*

mg/min	mL/hr
0.5	8
1	15
1.5	23
2	30
2.5	38
3	45
3.5	53
4	60
4.5	68
5	75
5.5	83
6	90

*Data from *The Criticare Drug Dose and Infusion Calculator Software*. Mt Vernon, Ill, Med-Pharm Information Systems, 1991.

Prostaglandin E₁, 500 μg in 250 mL (2 μg/mL)*†

Dose, μg/kg/min	Patient's Weight (lb/kg)																	
	2.2/1	4.4/2	6.6/3	8.8/4	11/5	22/10	33/15	44/20	55/25	66/30	77/35	88/40	99/45	110/50	121/55	132/60	143/65	154/70
	Infusion Rate, mL/hr																	
0.05	2	3	5	6	8	15	23	30	38	45	53	60	68	75	83	90	98	105
0.1	3	6	9	12	15	30	45	60	75	90	105	120	135	150	165	180	195	210
0.15	5	9	14	18	23	45	68	90	113	135	158	180	203	225	248	270	293	315
0.2	6	12	18	24	30	60	90	120	150	180	210	240	270	300	330	360	390	420
0.25	8	15	23	30	38	75	113	150	188	225	263	300	338	375	413	450	488	525
0.3	9	18	27	36	45	90	135	180	225	270	315	360	405	450	495	540	585	630
0.35	11	21	32	42	53	105	158	210	263	315	368	420	473	525	578	630	683	735
0.4	12	24	36	48	60	120	180	240	300	360	420	480	540	600	660	720	780	840

*Data from The Criticare Drug Dose and Infusion Calculator Software. Mt Vernon, Ill, Med-Pharm Information Systems, 1991.
†Infusion rate is found at intersection of "Dose" and Patient's Weight columns.

Propofol, Undiluted (10 mg/mL)*†

Dose, μg/kg/min	Patient's Weight (lb/kg)														
	65/30	77/35	88/40	99/45	110/50	121/55	132/60	143/65	154/70	165/75	176/80	187/85	198/90	209/95	220/100
	Infusion Rate, mL/hr														
100	18	21	24	27	30	33	36	39	42	45	48	51	54	57	60
110	20	23	26	30	33	36	40	43	46	50	53	56	59	63	66
120	22	25	29	32	36	40	43	47	50	54	58	61	65	68	72
130	23	27	31	35	39	43	47	51	55	59	62	66	70	74	78
140	25	29	34	38	42	46	50	55	59	63	67	71	76	80	84
150	27	32	36	41	45	50	54	59	63	68	72	77	81	86	90
160	29	34	38	43	48	53	58	62	67	72	77	82	86	91	96
170	31	36	41	46	51	56	61	66	71	77	82	87	92	97	102
180	32	38	43	49	54	59	65	70	76	81	86	92	97	103	108
190	34	40	46	51	57	63	68	74	80	86	91	97	103	108	114
200	36	42	48	54	60	66	72	78	84	90	96	102	108	114	120

*Data from The Criticare Drug Dose and Infusion Calculator Software. Mt Vernon, Ill, Med-Pharm Information Systems, 1991.
†Infusion rate is found at intersection of 'Dose' and Patient's Weight columns.

Sodium Nitroprusside, 50 mg in 250 mL (200 μg/mL)*†

Dose, μg/kg/min	66/30	77/35	88/40	99/45	110/50	121/55	132/60	143/65	154/70	165/75	176/80	187/85	198/90	209/95	220/100
							Infusion Rate, mL/hr								
0.1	1	1	1	1	2	2	2	2	2	2	2	3	3	3	3
0.2	2	2	2	3	3	3	4	4	4	5	5	5	5	6	6
0.3	3	3	4	4	5	5	5	6	6	7	7	8	8	9	9
0.4	4	4	5	5	6	7	7	8	8	9	10	10	11	11	12
0.5	5	5	6	7	8	8	9	10	11	11	12	13	14	14	15
0.6	5	6	7	8	8	10	11	12	13	14	14	15	16	17	18
0.7	6	7	8	10	11	12	13	14	15	16	17	18	19	20	21
0.8	7	8	10	11	12	13	14	16	17	18	19	20	22	23	24
0.9	8	10	11	12	14	15	16	18	19	20	22	23	24	26	27
1.0	9	11	12	14	15	17	18	20	21	23	24	26	27	29	30
2.0	18	21	24	27	30	33	36	39	42	45	48	51	54	57	60
3.0	27	32	36	41	45	50	54	59	63	68	72	77	81	86	90
4.0	36	42	48	54	60	66	72	78	84	90	96	102	108	114	120
5.0	45	53	60	68	75	83	90	98	105	113	120	128	135	143	150
6.0	54	63	72	81	90	99	108	117	126	135	144	153	162	171	180
7.0	63	74	84	95	105	116	126	137	147	158	168	179	189	200	210
8.0	72	84	96	108	120	132	144	156	168	180	192	204	216	228	240
9.0	81	95	108	122	135	149	162	176	189	203	216	230	243	257	270
10	90	105	120	135	150	165	180	195	210	225	240	255	270	285	300

Patient's Weight (lb/kg)

*Data from The Criticare Drug Dose and Infusion Calculator Software. Mt Vernon, Ill, Med-Pharm Information Systems, 1991.
†Infusion rate is found at intersection of "Dose" and Patient's Weight columns.

Succinylcholine, 250 mg in 250
mL (1 mg/mL)*

mg/min	mL/hr
0.5	30
1	60
2	120
3	180
4	240
5	300
6	360
7	420
8	480
9	540
10	600

*Data from *The Criticare Drug Dose and Infusion Calculator Software.* Mt Vernon, Ill, Med-Pharm Information Systems, 1991.

Epidural Sufentanil, 100 μg in 100
mL (1 μg/mL)*

μg/hr	mL/hr
5	5
10	10
15	15
20	20
25	25
30	30

*Data from *The Criticare Drug Dose and Infusion Calculator Software.* Mt Vernon, Ill, Med-Pharm Information Systems, 1991.

Intravenous Sufentanil, 500 µg in 100 mL (5 µg/mL)*†

Patient's Weight $\left(\dfrac{\text{lb}}{\text{kg}}\right)$

Dose, µg/kg/min	$\frac{66}{30}$	$\frac{77}{35}$	$\frac{88}{40}$	$\frac{99}{45}$	$\frac{110}{50}$	$\frac{121}{55}$	$\frac{132}{60}$	$\frac{143}{65}$	$\frac{154}{70}$	$\frac{165}{75}$	$\frac{176}{80}$	$\frac{187}{85}$	$\frac{198}{90}$	$\frac{209}{95}$	$\frac{220}{100}$
							Infusion Rate, mL/hr								
0.01	4	4	5	5	6	7	7	8	8	9	10	10	11	11	12
0.02	7	8	10	11	12	13	14	16	17	18	19	20	22	23	24
0.03	11	13	14	16	18	20	22	23	25	27	29	31	32	34	36
0.04	14	17	19	22	24	26	29	31	34	36	38	41	43	46	48
0.05	18	21	24	27	30	33	36	39	42	45	48	51	54	57	60

*Data from: The Criticare Drug Dose and Infusion Calculator Software. Mt Vernon, Ill, Med-Pharm Information Systems, 1991.
†Infusion rate is found at intersection of "Dose" and Patient's Weight columns.

Trimetaphan, 1500 mg in 500 mL
(3 mg/mL)*

mg/min	mL/hr
0.3	6
0.4	8
0.5	10
0.6	12
0.7	14
0.8	16
0.9	18
1	20
1.5	30
2	40
2.5	50
3	60
3.5	70
4	80
4.5	90
5	100
5.5	110
6	120

*Data from *The Criticare Drug Dose and Infusion Calculator Software*. Mt Vernon, Ill, Med-Pharm Information Systems, 1991.

Vasopressin, 200 Units in 250 mL
(0.8 Units/mL)*

Units/min	mL/hr
0.2	15
0.3	23
0.4	30
0.5	38
0.6	45
0.7	53
0.8	60
0.9	68
1	75

*Data from *The Criticare Drug Dose and Infusion Calculator Software*. Mt Vernon, Ill, Med-Pharm Information Systems, 1991.

Vecuronium, 20 mg in 100 mL (0.2 mg/mL)*†

Dose, μg/kg/min	Patient's Weight (lb/kg)														
	66/30	77/35	88/40	99/45	110/50	121/55	132/60	143/65	154/70	165/75	176/80	187/85	198/90	209/95	220/100
	Infusion Rate, mL/hr														
1	9	11	12	14	15	17	18	20	21	23	24	26	27	29	30
1.1	10	12	13	15	17	18	20	21	23	25	26	28	30	31	33
1.2	11	13	14	16	18	20	22	23	25	27	29	31	32	34	36
1.3	12	14	16	18	20	21	23	25	27	29	31	33	35	37	39
1.4	13	15	17	19	21	23	25	27	29	32	34	36	38	40	42
1.5	14	16	18	20	23	25	27	29	32	34	36	38	41	43	45
1.6	14	17	19	22	24	26	29	31	33	36	38	41	43	46	48
1.7	15	18	20	23	26	28	31	33	36	38	41	43	46	48	51
1.8	16	19	22	24	27	30	32	35	38	41	43	46	49	51	54
1.9	17	20	23	26	29	31	34	37	40	43	46	48	51	54	57
2	18	21	24	27	30	33	36	39	42	45	48	51	54	57	60

*Data from The Criticare Drug Dose and Infusion Calculator Software. Mt Vernon, Ill, Med-Pharm Information Systems, 1991.
†Infusion rate is found at intersection of "Dose" and Patient's Weight columns.

Appendix E

TRADE NAME TABLE

Trade names listed represent examples chosen by the author and are not complete lists of marketed drugs.

Trade Name	Generic Name
Adalat	Nifedipine
Adenocard	Adenosine
Adrenaline	Epinephrine HCl
Aldomet	Methyldopa
Alfenta	Alfentanil HCl
Americaine	Benzocaine
Amicar	Aminocaproic acid
Amidate	Etomidate
Aminophylline	Aminophylline
Anectine	Succinylcholine chloride
Antilirium	Physostigmine salicylate
Apresoline	Hydralazine HCl
Aquamephyton	Phytonadione — vitamin K
Arduan	Pipecuronium bromide
Arfonad	Trimethaphan camsylate
Astramorph	Morphine sulfate
Ativan	Lorazepam
Atropine sulfate	Atropine sulfate
Benadryl	Diphenhydramine HCl
Bicitra	Sodium citrate
Brethaire	Terbutaline sulfate
Bretylol	Bretylium tosylate
Brevibloc	Esmolol HCl
Brevital	Methohexital sodium
Bricanyl	Terbutaline sulfate
Calan	Verapamil HCl
Calcium chloride	Calcium chloride
Calcium gluconate	Calcium gluconate
Capoten	Captopril
Carbocaine	Mepivacaine HCl
Carfin	Warfarin sodium
Catapres	Clonidine HCl
Citanest	Prilocaine HCl
Cocaine Hcl	Cocaine HCl
Compazine	Prochlorperazine
Cordarone	Amiodarone
Coumadin	Warfarin sodium
Dalmane	Flurazepam HCl
Dantrium	Dantrolene sodium
DDAVP	Desmopressin acetate
Decadron	Dexamethasone
Demerol	Meperidine HCl

(Continued.)

Trade Name	Generic Name
Dermoplast	Benzocaine
Dilantin	Phenytoin sodium
Dilaudid	Hydromorphone HCl
Dilaudid HP	Hydromorphone HCl
Diprivan	Propofol
Dobutrex	Dobutamine HCl
Dolophine	Methadone HCl
Dopram	Doxapram HCl
Duramorph	Morphine sulfate
Duranest	Etidocaine HCl
Edecrin	Ethacrynic acid
Enlon	Edrophonium chloride
Ephedrine sulfate	Ephedrine sulfate
Epinephrine	Epinephrine HCl
Ergotrate	Ergonovine maleate
Ethrane	Enflurane
Flaxedil	Gallamine triethiodide
Fluothane	Halothane
Forane	Isoflurane
Glucagon	Glucagon
Haldol	Haloperidol
Halperon	Haloperidol
Heparin sodium	Heparin sodium
Hespan	Hetastarch
Hexadrol	Dexamethasone
Hurricaine	Benzocaine
Hydrocortisone acetate	Hydrocortisone
Hydrocortisone cypionate	Hydrocortisone
Hydrocortisone sodium succinate	Hydrocortisone
Hydrocortisone sodium phosphate	Hydrocortisone
Inapsine	Droperidol
Inderal	Propranolol HCl
Infumorph	Morphine sulfate
Inocor	Amrinone lactate
Intropin	Dopamine HCl
Isoptin	Verapamil HCl
Isuprel	Isoproterenol HCl
Ketalar	Ketamine HCl
Konakion	Phytonadione—vitamin K
Lanoxin	Digoxin
Lasix	Furosemide
Levophed	Norepinephrine bitartrate

Librium	Chlordiazepoxide HCl
Lopressor	Metoprolol tartrate
Magnesium sulfate	Magnesium sulfate
Marcaine	Bupivacaine HCl
Mazicon	Flumazenil
Medihaler-ISO	Isoproterenol HCl
Medrol	Methylprednisolone
Mestinon	Pyridostigmine bromide
Methergine	Methylergonovine maleate
Methyldopate	Methyldopa
Metubine iodide	Metocurine iodide
Mivacron	Mivacurium chloride
Morphine	Morphine sulfate
MS contin	Morphine sulfate
Narcan	Naloxone HCl
Neosynephrine	Phenylephrine HCl
Nesacaine	Chloroprocaine HCl
Nipride	Sodium nitroprusside
Nitro-Bid	Nitroglycerin
Nitrocine	Nitroglycerin
Nitrodisc	Nitroglycerin
Nitrogard	Nitroglycerin
Nitroglyn	Nitroglycerin
Nitrol	Nitroglycerin
Nitrolin	Nitroglycerin
Nitrong	Nitroglycerin
Nitropress	Sodium nitroprusside
Nitrostat	Nitroglycerin
Nitrous oxide	Nitrous oxide
Norcuron	Vecuronium bromide
Normodyne	Labetalol HCl
Novocaine	Procaine HCl
Nubain	Nalbuphine HCl
Nuromax	Doxacurium chloride
Osmitrol	Mannitol
Panwarfin	Warfarin sodium
Pavulon	Pancuronium
Pentothal	Thiopental sodium
Pepcid	Famotidine
Phenergan	Promethazine HCl
Pitocin	Oxytocin
Pitressin	Vasopressin
Polocaine	Mepivacaine HCl
Pontocaine	Tetracaine

(Continued.)

Trade Name	Generic Name
Potassium chloride	Potassium chloride
Procan SR	Procainamide HCl
Procardia	Nifedipine
Pronestyl	Procainamide HCl
Prostigmine	Neostigmine
Prostin VR	Prostaglandin E_1—alprostadil
Protamine sulfate	Protamine sulfate
Quelicin	Succinylcholine chloride
Regitine	Phentolamine
Reglan	Metoclopramide
Regonal	Pyridostigmine bromide
Reversol	Edrophonium chloride
Rhulicaine	Benzocaine
Robinul	Glycopyrrolate
Sandimmune	Cyclosporine
Scopolamine HBr	Scopolamine hydrobromide
Seconal	Secobarbital
Sensorcaine	Bupivacaine HCl
Servoflurane	Servoflurane
Shohl's Solution	Sodium citrate
Sodium bicarbonate	Sodium bicarbonate
Sofarin	Warfarin sodium
Solarcaine	Benzocaine
Solu-Cortef	Hydrocortisone
Solu-Medrol	Methylprednisolone sodium succinate
Stadol	Butorphanol tartrate
Stimate	Desmopressin acetate
Sublimaze	Fentanyl
Sucostrin	Succinylcholine chloride
Sufenta	Sufentanil citrate
Suprane	Desflurane
Syntocinon	Oxytocin
Tagamet	Cimetidine
Tambocor	Flecainide acetate
Tenormin	Atenolol
Tensilon	Edrophonium chloride
Thorazine	Chlorpromazine HCl
Toradol	Ketorolac
Tracrium	Atracurium besylate
Trandate	Labetalol HCl
Transderm-Nitro	Nitroglycerin
Tridil	Nitroglycerin

Tubocurarine chloride	D-Tubocurarine chloride
Urolene blue	Methylene blue
Valium	Diazepam
Vasoxyl	Methoxamine HCl
Versed	Midazolam
Wyamine	Mephentermine Sulfate
Xylocaine	Lidocaine HCl
Yutopar	Ritodrine HCl
Zantac	Ranitidine

Index

A

Abdomen
  cramps in
    from propofol, 173
    from pyridostigmine, 180
    from vasopressin, 204
  discomfort in
    from cyclosporine, 41
    from ethacrynic acid, 69
    from verapamil, 208
  pain in
    from amrinone, 10
    from bretylium, 17
    from captopril, 27
    from desmopressin acetate, 45
    from flecainide, 76
    from flurazepam, 80
    from methylene blue, 122
    from nitroglycerin, 144
    from potassium chloride, 162
Abortion, spontaneous/threatened,
    ritodrine for, 181–183
Abscess(es)
  from calcium chloride, 23
  from calcium gluconate, 25
  from cyclosporine, 41
  necrotic, of skin, from
    methylene blue, 122
  from potassium chloride, 163
Accommodation, impaired, from
    scopolamine, 184
ACE inhibitors, interaction of
  with nifedipine, 141
  with potassium chloride, 161
  with verapamil, 207

Acetaminophen, interactions of
    metoclopramide with,
    126
Acetazolamide, interaction of
    cyclosporine with, 40
Acidosis
  central venous, from sodium
    bicarbonate, 189
  cerebrospinal fluid, from sodium
    bicarbonate, 189
  intracellular, from sodium
    bicarbonate, 189
  from mannitol, 110
  metabolic (see Metabolic
    acidosis)
  respiratory (see Respiratory
    acidosis)
Acid pulmonary aspiration,
    prophylaxis against
  cimetidine for, 32–33
  famotidine for, 73
  ranitidine for, 180–181
Acid taste from midazolam, 131
Acyclovir, interaction of
    cyclosporine with, 40
Adalat, 140–142
Adams-Stokes seizures,
    paradoxical precipitation
    of, from isoproterenol,
    97
Adenocard, 1–3
Adenosine, 1–3
Adrenaline, 63–65
Adrenergic blocking drugs,
    peripheral, interaction of
    furosemide with, 82

Zofran®
(ondansetron hydrochloride)
Injection

For IV Injection Only

DESCRIPTION: The active ingredient in Zofran® Injection is ondansetron hydrochloride (HCl), the racemic form of ondansetron and a selective blocking agent of the serotonin 5-HT$_3$ receptor type. Chemically it is (±) 1, 2, 3, 9-tetrahydro-9-methyl-3-[(2-methyl-1H-imidazol-1-yl)methyl]-4H-carbazol-4-one, monohydrochloride, dihydrate. It has the following structural formula:

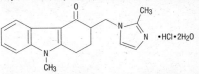

The empirical formula is $C_{18}H_{19}N_3O \cdot HCl \cdot 2H_2O$, representing a molecular weight of 365.9.
Ondansetron HCl is a white to off-white powder that is soluble in water and normal saline.
Zofran Injection is a clear, colorless, nonpyrogenic, sterile solution for intravenous (IV) injection.

Each 1 mL of aqueous solution in the 2-mL single-dose vial contains 2 mg of ondansetron as the hydrochloride dihydrate; 9.0 mg of sodium chloride, USP; and 0.5 mg of citric acid monohydrate, USP and 0.25 mg of sodium citrate dihydrate, USP as buffers in water for injection, USP.

Each 1 mL of aqueous solution in the 20-mL multidose vial contains 2 mg of ondansetron as the hydrochloride dihydrate; 8.3 mg of sodium chloride, USP; 0.5 mg of citric acid monohydrate, USP and 0.25 mg of sodium citrate dihydrate, USP as buffers; and 1.2 mg of methylparaben, NF and 0.15 mg of propylparaben, NF as preservatives in water for injection, USP. The pH of the injection solution is 3.3 to 4.0.

CLINICAL PHARMACOLOGY:
Pharmacodynamics: Ondansetron is a selective 5-HT$_3$ receptor antagonist. While ondansetron's mechanism of action has not been fully characterized, it is not a dopamine-receptor antagonist. Serotonin receptors of the 5-HT$_3$ type are present both peripherally on vagal nerve terminals and centrally in the chemoreceptor trigger zone of the area postrema. It is not certain whether ondansetron's antiemetic action in chemotherapy-induced emesis is mediated centrally, peripherally, or in both sites. However, cytotoxic chemotherapy appears to be associated with release of serotonin from the enterochromaffin cells of the small intestine. In humans, urinary 5-HIAA (5-hydroxyindoleacetic acid) excretion increases after cisplatin administration in parallel with the onset of emesis. The released serotonin may stimulate the vagal afferents through the 5-HT$_3$ receptors and initiate the vomiting reflex.

In animals, the emetic response to cisplatin can be prevented by pretreatment with an inhibitor of serotonin synthesis, bilateral abdominal vagotomy and greater splanchnic nerve section, or pretreatment with a serotonin 5-HT$_3$ receptor antagonist.

In normal volunteers, single IV doses of 0.15 mg/kg of ondansetron had no effect on esophageal motility, gastric motility, lower esophageal sphincter pressure, or small intestinal transit time. In another study in six normal male volunteers, a 16-mg dose infused over 5 minutes showed no effect of the drug on cardiac output, heart rate, stroke volume, blood pressure, or electrocardiogram (ECG). Multiday administration of ondansetron has been shown to slow colonic transit in normal volunteers. Ondansetron has no effect on plasma prolactin concentrations.

Ondansetron does not alter the respiratory depressant effects produced by alfentanil or the degree of neuromuscular blockade produced by atracurium. Interactions with general or local anesthetics have not been studied.

Pharmacokinetics: Ondansetron is extensively metabolized in humans, with approximately 5% of a radiolabeled dose recovered as the parent compound from the urine. The primary metabolic pathway is hydroxylation on the indole ring followed by glucuronide or sulfate conjugation.

In normal volunteers, the following mean pharmacokinetic data have been determined following a single 0.15-mg/kg IV dose.

Pharmacokinetics in Normal Volunteers

Age-group	n	Peak Plasma Concentration (ng/mL)	Mean Elimination Half-life (h)	Plasma Clearance (L/h/kg)
19-40	11	102	3.5	0.381
61-74	12	106	4.7	0.319
≥ 75	11	170	5.5	0.262

From a single-dose infusion study, patients with severe hepatic impairment showed a five-fold and those with mild-to-moderate liver impairment a two-fold reduction in mean plasma clearance, with increases in the mean apparent volume of distribution of less than two-fold, as compared to normals. The mean half-life of 3.6 hours in normals increased to 9.2 hours in patients with mild-to-moderate hepatic impairment and was prolonged to 20.6 hours in patients with severe hepatic insufficiency.

A reduction in clearance and increase in elimination half-life are seen in patients over 75 years old. In clinical trials with patients with cancer, there was neither a difference in safety nor efficacy between patients over 65 years of age and those under 65 years of age; there was an insufficient number of patients over 75 years of age to permit conclusions in that age-group. No adjustment in dosage is recommended in the elderly.

In adult cancer patients, the mean elimination half-life was 4.0 hours, and there was no difference in the multidose pharmacokinetics over a 4-day period. In a study of 21 pediatric cancer patients (aged 4 to 18 years) who received three IV doses of 0.15 mg/kg of ondansetron at 4-hour intervals, patients older than 15 years of age exhibited ondansetron pharmacokinetic parameters similar to those of adults. Patients aged 4 to 12 years generally showed higher clearance and somewhat larger volume of distribution than adults. Most pediatric patients younger than 15 years of age with cancer had a shorter (2.4 hours)ondansetron plasma half-life than patients older than 15 years of age. It is not known whether these differences in ondansetron plasma half-life may result in differences in efficacy between adults and some young children (see CLINICAL TRIALS: Pediatric Studies).

In normal volunteers (19 to 39 years old, n=23), the peak plasma concentration was 264 ng/mL following a single 32-mg dose administered as a 15-minute IV infusion. The mean elimination half-life was 4.1 hours. Systemic exposure to 32 mg of ondansetron was not proportional to dose as measured by comparing dose-normalized AUC values to an 8-mg dose. This is consistent with a small decrease in systemic clearance with increasing plasma concentrations.

Plasma protein binding of ondansetron as measured in vitro was 70% to 76%, with binding constant over the pharmacologic concentration range (10 to 500 ng/mL). Circulating drug also distributes into erythrocytes.

A positive lymphoblast transformation test to ondansetron has been reported, which suggests immunologic sensitivity to ondansetron.

Zofran® (ondansetron hydrochloride) Injection

CLINICAL TRIALS:

Chemotherapy-Induced Nausea and Vomiting: In a double-blind study of three different dosing regimens of Zofran® Injection, 0.015 mg/kg, 0.15 mg/kg, and 0.30 mg/kg, each given three times during the course of cancer chemotherapy, the 0.15-mg/kg dosing regimen was more effective than the 0.015-mg/kg dosing regimen. The 0.30-mg/kg dosing regimen was not shown to be more effective than the 0.15-mg/kg dosing regimen.

Cisplatin-Based Chemotherapy: In a double-blind study in 28 patients, Zofran Injection (three 0.15-mg/kg doses) was significantly more effective than placebo in preventing nausea and vomiting induced by cisplatin-based chemotherapy. Treatment response was as follows:

Prevention of Chemotherapy-Induced Nausea and Emesis in Single-Day Cisplatin Therapy*

	Zofran Injection	Placebo	p Value[†]
Number of patients	14	14	
Treatment response			
0 Emetic episodes	2 (14%)	0 (0%)	
1-2 Emetic episodes	8 (57%)	0 (0%)	
3-5 Emetic episodes	2 (14%)	1 (7%)	
More than 5 emetic episodes/rescued	2 (14%)	13 (93%)	0.001
Median number of emetic episodes	1.5	Undefined[‡]	
Median time to first emetic episode (h)	11.6	2.8	0.001
Median nausea scores (0-100)[§]	3	59	0.034
Global satisfaction with control of nausea and vomiting (0-100)[‖]	96	10.5	0.009

*Chemotherapy was high dose (100 and 120 mg/m^2; Zofran Injection n=6, placebo n=5) or moderate dose (50 and 80 mg/m^2; Zofran Injection n=8, placebo n=9). Other chemotherapeutic agents included fluorouracil, doxorubicin, and cyclophosphamide. There was no difference between treatments in the types of chemotherapy that would account for differences in response.
[†] Efficacy based on "all patients treated" analysis.
[‡] Median undefined since at least 50% of the patients were rescued or had more than five emetic episodes.
[§] Visual analog scale assessment of nausea: 0=no nausea, 100=nausea as bad as it can be.
[‖] Visual analog scale assessment of satisfaction: 0=not at all satisfied, 100=totally satisfied.

Ondansetron was compared with metoclopramide in a single-blind trial in 307 patients receiving cisplatin $\geq$ 100 mg/m^2 with or without other chemotherapeutic agents. Patients received the first dose of ondansetron or metoclopramide 30 minutes before cisplatin. Two additional ondansetron doses were administered 4 and 8 hours later, or five additional metoclopramide doses were administered 2, 4, 7, 10, and 13 hours later. Cisplatin was administered over a period of 3 hours or less. Episodes of vomiting and retching were tabulated over the period of 24 hours after cisplatin. The results of this study are summarized below:

Prevention of Emesis Induced by Cisplatin (≥100 mg/m²) Single-Day Therapy*

	Zofran Injection	Metoclopramide	p Value
Dose	0.15 mg/kg x 3	2 mg/kg x 6	
Number of patients in efficacy population	136	133	
Treatment response			
0 Emetic episodes	54 (40%)	41 (30%)	
1-2 Emetic episodes	34 (25%)	30 (22%)	
3-5 Emetic episodes	19 (14%)	18 (13%)	
More than 5 emetic episodes/rescued	29 (21%)	49 (36%)	
Comparison of treatments with respect to			
0 Emetic episodes	54/136	41/138	0.083
More than 5 emetic episodes/rescued	29/136	49/138	0.009
Median number of emetic episodes	1	2	0.005
Median time to first emetic episode (h)	20.5	4.3	<0.001
Global satisfaction with control of nausea and vomiting (0-100)†	85	63	0.001
Acute dystonic reactions	0	8	0.005
Akathisia	0	10	0.002

*In addition to cisplatin, 68% of patients received other chemotherapeutic agents, including cyclophosphamide, etoposide, and fluorouracil. There was no difference between treatments in the types of chemotherapy that would account for differences in response.

† Visual analog scale assessment: 0=not at all satisfied, 100=totally satisfied.

Forty-one of the ondansetron patients were over 65 years of age. The complete response rate (zero emetic episodes) was 41% in this group compared with 40% in those 65 years old or younger.

In a stratified, randomized, double-blind, parallel-group, multicenter study, a single 32-mg dose of ondansetron was compared with three 0.15-mg/kg doses in patients receiving cisplatin doses of either 50 to 70 mg/m² or ≥100 mg/m². Patients received the first ondansetron dose 30 minutes before cisplatin. Two additional ondansetron doses were administered 4 and 8 hours later to the group receiving three 0.15-mg/kg doses. In both strata, significantly fewer patients on the single 32-mg dose than those receiving the three-dose regimen failed.

Prevention of Chemotherapy-Induced Nausea and Emesis in Single-Dose Therapy

	Ondansetron Dose		p Value
	0.15 mg/kg x 3	32 mg x 1	
High-dose cisplatin (≥100 mg/m²)			
Number of patients	100	102	
Treatment response			
0 Emetic episodes	41 (41%)	49 (48%)	0.315
1-2 Emetic episodes	19 (19%)	25 (25%)	
3-5 Emetic episodes	4 (4%)	8 (8%)	
More than 5 emetic episodes/rescued	36 (36%)	20 (20%)	0.009

ofran® (ondansetron hydrochloride) Injection

Prevention of Chemotherapy-Induced Nausea and Emesis in Single-Dose Therapy

| | Ondansetron Dose | | |
	0.15 mg/kg x 3	32 mg x 1	p Value
Median time to first emetic episode (h)	21.7	23	0.173
Median nausea scores (0-100)*	28	13	0.004
Medium-dose cisplatin (50-70 mg/m²)			
Number of patients	101	93	
Treatment response			
0 Emetic episodes	62 (61%)	68 (73%)	0.083
1-2 Emetic episodes	11 (11%)	14 (15%)	
3-5 Emetic episodes	6 (6%)	3 (3%)	
More than 5 emetic episodes/rescued	22 (22%)	8 (9%)	0.011
Median time to first emetic episode (h)	Undefined†	Undefined	0.084
Median nausea scores (0-100)*	9	3	0.131

*Visual analog scale assessment: 0=no nausea, 100=nausea as bad as it can be.
† Median undefined since at least 50% of patients did not have any emetic episodes.

Cyclophosphamide-Based Chemotherapy: In a double-blind, placebo-controlled study of Zofran Injection (three 0.15-mg/kg doses) in 20 patients receiving cyclophosphamide (500 to 600 mg/m²) chemotherapy, Zofran Injection was significantly more effective than placebo in preventing nausea and vomiting. The results are summarized below:

Prevention of Chemotherapy-Induced Nausea and Emesis in Single-Day Cyclophosphamide Therapy*

	Zofran Injection	Placebo	p Value†
Number of patients	10	10	
Treatment response			
0 Emetic episodes	7 (70%)	0 (0%)	0.001
1-2 Emetic episodes	0 (0%)	2 (20%)	
3-5 Emetic episodes	2 (20%)	4 (40%)	
More than 5 emetic episodes/rescued	1 (10%)	4 (40%)	0.131
Median number of emetic episodes	0	4	0.008
Median time to first emetic episode (h)	Undefined‡	8.79	
Median nausea scores (0-100)§	0	60	0.001
Global satisfaction with control of nausea and vomiting (0-100)‖	100	52	0.008

Zofran® (ondansetron hydrochloride) Injection

*Chemotherapy consisted of cyclophosphamide in all patients, plus other agents, including fluorouracil, doxorubicin, methotrexate, and vincristine. There was no difference between treatments in the type of chemotherapy that would account for differences in response.

† Efficacy based on "all patients treated" analysis.

‡Median undefined since at least 50% of patients did not have any emetic episodes.

§ Visual analog scale assessment of nausea: 0=no nausea, 100=nausea as bad as it can be.

‖ Visual analog scale assessment of satisfaction: 0=not at all satisfied, 100=totally satisfied.

Retreatment: In uncontrolled trials, 127 patients receiving cisplatin (median dose, 100 mg/m²) and ondansetron who had two or fewer emetic episodes were retreated with ondansetron and chemotherapy, mainly cisplatin, for a total of 269 retreatment courses (median, 2; range, 1 to 10). No emetic episodes occurred in 160 (59%), and two or fewer emetic episodes occurred in 217 (81%) retreatment courses.

Pediatric Studies: Four open-label, noncomparative (one US, three foreign) trials have been performed with 209 pediatric cancer patients aged 4 to 18 years given a variety of cisplatin or non-cisplatin regimens. In the three foreign trials, the initial Zofran Injection dose ranged from 0.04 to 0.87 mg/kg for a total dose of 2.16 to 12 mg. This was followed by the oral administration of ondansetron ranging from 4 to 24 mg daily for 3 days. In the US trial, Zofran was administered intravenously (only) in three doses of 0.15 mg/kg each for a total daily dose of 7.2 to 39 mg. In these studies, 58% of the 196 evaluable patients had a complete response (no emetic episodes) on day 1. Thus, prevention of emesis in these children was essentially the same as for patients older than 18 years of age. Overall, Zofran Injection was well tolerated in these pediatric patients.

Postoperative Nausea and Vomiting: *Prevention of Postoperative Nausea and Vomiting:* Surgical patients who received ondansetron immediately before the induction of general balanced anesthesia (barbiturate: thiopental, methohexital or thiamylal; opioid: alfentanil or fentanyl; nitrous oxide; neuro-muscular blockade: succinylcholine/curare and/or vecuronium or atracurium; and supplemental isoflurane) were evaluated in two double-blind US studies involving 554 patients. Zofran Injection (4 mg) IV given over 2 to 5 minutes was significantly more effective than placebo. The results of these studies are summarized below:

Prevention of Postoperative Nausea and Vomiting

	Ondansetron 4 mg IV	Placebo	p Value
Study 1			
Emetic episodes:			
Number of patients	136	139	
Treatment response over 24-hr postoperative period			
0 Emetic episodes	103 (76%)	64 (46%)	<0.001
1 Emetic episode	13 (10%)	17 (12%)	
More than 1 emetic episode/rescued	20 (15%)	58 (42%)	
Nausea assessments:			
Number of patients	134	136	
No nausea over 24-hr postoperative period	56 (42%)	39 (29%)	

Zofran® (ondansetron hydrochloride) Injection

Prevention of Postoperative Nausea and Vomiting

	Ondansetron 4 mg IV	Placebo	p Value
Study 2			
Emetic episodes:			
Number of patients	136	143	
Treatment response over			
24-hr postoperative period			
0 Emetic episodes	85 (63%)	63 (44%)	0.002
1 Emetic episode	16 (12%)	29 (20%)	
More than 1 emetic			
episode/rescued	35 (26%)	51 (36%)	
Nausea assessments:			
Number of patients	125	133	
No nausea over 24-hr			
postoperative period	48 (38%)	42 (32%)	

The study populations in all trials thus far consisted of mainly women undergoing laparoscopic procedures. While some men were included in some trials with similar results, clearance of the drug is more rapid in men and sufficient numbers of men have not been clinically studied to be certain that efficacy and safety have been established. Few patients undergoing major abdominal surgery have been studied.

Prevention of Further Postoperative Nausea and Vomiting: Surgical patients receiving general balanced anesthesia (barbiturate: thiopental, methohexital or thiamylal; opioid: alfentanil or fentanyl; nitrous oxide; neuromuscular blockade: succinylcholine/curare and/or vecuronium or atracurium; and supplemental isoflurane) who received no prophylactic antiemetics and who experienced nausea and/or vomiting within 2 hours postoperatively were evaluated in two double-blind US studies involving 441 patients. Patients who experienced an episode of postoperative nausea and/or vomiting were given Zofran Injection (4 mg) IV over 2 to 5 minutes, and this was significantly more effective than placebo. The results of these studies are summarized below:

Prevention of Further Postoperative Nausea and Vomiting

	Ondansetron 4 mg IV	Placebo	p Value
Study 1			
Emetic episodes:			
Number of patients	104	117	
Treatment response			
24 hrs after study drug			
0 Emetic episodes	49 (47%)	19 (16%)	<0.001
1 Emetic episode	12 (12%)	9 (8%)	
More than 1 emetic			
episode/rescued	43 (41%)	89 (76%)	
Median time to first			
emetic episode (min)*	55.0	43.0	
Nausea assessments:			
Number of patients	98	102	
Mean nausea score over			
24-hr postoperative period†	1.7	3.1	

Prevention of Further Postoperative Nausea and Vomiting

	Ondansetron 4 mg IV	Placebo	p Value
Study 2			
Emetic episodes:			
Number of patients	112	108	
Treatment response			
24 hrs after study drug			
0 Emetic episodes	49 (44%)	28 (26%)	0.006
1 Emetic episode	14 (13%)	3 (3%)	
More than 1 emetic			
episode/rescued	49 (44%)	77 (71%)	
Median time to first			
emetic episode (min)*	60.5	34.0	
Nausea assessments:			
Number of patients	105	85	
Mean nausea score over			
24-hr postoperative period†	1.9	2.9	

*After administration of study drug.
†Nausea measured on a scale of 0-10 with 0=no nausea, 10=nausea as bad as it can be.

The study populations in all trials thus far consisted of mainly women undergoing laparoscopic procedures. While some men were included in some trials with similar results, clearance of the drug is more rapid in men and sufficient numbers of men have not been clinically studied to be certain that efficacy and safety have been established. Few patients undergoing major abdominal surgery have been studied.

INDICATIONS AND USAGE:

1. Prevention of nausea and vomiting associated with initial and repeat courses of emetogenic cancer chemotherapy, including high-dose cisplatin. Efficacy of the 32-mg single dose beyond 24 hours in these patients has not been established.

2. Prevention of postoperative nausea and/or vomiting. As with other antiemetics, routine prophylaxis is not recommended for patients in whom there is little expectation that nausea and/or vomiting will occur perioperatively. In patients where nausea and/or vomiting must be avoided postoperatively, Zofran® Injection is recommended even where the incidence of postoperative nausea and/or vomiting is low. For patients who have nausea and/or vomiting postoperatively, Zofran Injection may be given to prevent further episodes (see CLINICAL TRIALS).

CONTRAINDICATIONS: Zofran® Injection is contraindicated for patients known to have hypersensitivity to the drug.

PRECAUTIONS: Ondansetron is not a drug that stimulates gastric or intestinal peristalsis. It should not be used instead of nasogastric suction. As with other antiemetics, the use of ondansetron in abdominal surgery may mask a progressive ileus and/or gastric distension.

Drug Interactions: Ondansetron does not itself appear to induce or inhibit the cytochrome P-450 drug-metabolizing enzyme system of the liver. Because ondansetron is metabolized by hepatic cytochrome P-450 drug-metabolizing enzymes, inducers or inhibitors of these enzymes may change the clearance and, hence, the half-life of ondansetron. On the basis of limited available data, no dosage adjustment is recommended for patients on these drugs. Tumor response to chemotherapy in the P 388 mouse leukemia model is not affected by ondansetron. In humans, carmustine, etoposide, and cisplatin do not affect the pharmacokinetics of ondansetron.

Zofran® (ondansetron hydrochloride) Injection

Carcinogenesis, Mutagenesis, Impairment of Fertility: Carcinogenic effects were not seen in 2-year studies in rats and mice with oral ondansetron doses up to 10 and 30 mg/kg per day, respectively. Ondansetron was not mutagenic in standard tests for mutagenicity. Oral administration of ondansetron up to 15 mg/kg per day did not affect fertility or general reproductive performance of male and female rats.

Pregnancy: *Teratogenic Effects: Pregnancy Category B:* Reproduction studies have been performed in pregnant rats and rabbits at IV doses up to 4 mg/kg per day and have revealed no evidence of impaired fertility or harm to the fetus due to ondansetron. There are, however, no adequate and well-controlled studies in pregnant women. Because animal reproduction studies are not always predictive of human response, this drug should be used during pregnancy only if clearly needed.

Nursing Mothers: Ondansetron is excreted in the breast milk of rats. It is not known whether ondansetron is excreted in human milk. Because many drugs are excreted in human milk, caution should be exercised when ondansetron is administered to a nursing woman.

Pediatric Use: Little information is available about dosage in children 3 years of age or younger (see DOSAGE AND ADMINISTRATION section for use in children 4 to 18 years of age receiving cancer chemotherapy).

Use in Elderly Patients: Dosage adjustment is not needed in patients over the age of 65 (see CLINICAL PHARMACOLOGY). Prevention of nausea and vomiting in elderly patients was no different than in younger age-groups.

ADVERSE REACTIONS:

Chemotherapy-Induced Nausea and Vomiting: The following adverse events have been reported in individuals receiving ondansetron at a dosage of three 0.15-mg/kg doses or as a single 32-mg dose in clinical trials. These patients were receiving concomitant chemotherapy, primarily cisplatin, and IV fluids. Most were receiving a diuretic.

Principal Adverse Events in Comparative Trials

	Number of Patients With Event			
	Zofran® Injection 0.15 mg/kg x 3 n=419	Zofran Injection 32 mg x 1 n=220	Metoclopramide n=156	Placebo n=34
Diarrhea	16%	8%	44%	18%
Headache	17%	25%	7%	15%
Fever	8%	7%	5%	3%
Akathisia	0%	0%	6%	0%
Acute dystonic reactions*	0%	0%	5%	0%

*See Central Nervous System below.

The following have been reported during controlled clinical trials or in the routine management of patients. The percentage figures are based on clinical trial experience.

Gastrointestinal: Constipation has been reported in 11% of chemotherapy patients receiving multiday ondansetron.

Hepatic: In comparative trials in cisplatin chemotherapy patients with normal baseline values of aspartate transaminase (AST) and alanine transaminase (ALT), these enzymes have been reported to exceed twice the upper limit of normal in approximately 5% of patients. The increases were transient and did not appear to be related to dose or duration of therapy. On repeat exposure, similar transient elevations in transaminase values occurred in some courses, but symptomatic hepatic disease did not occur.

There have been reports of liver failure and death in patients with cancer receiving concurrent medications including potentially hepatotoxic cytotoxic chemotherapy and antibiotics. The etiology of the liver failure is unclear.

Integumentary: Rash has occurred in approximately 1% of patients receiving ondansetron.

Central Nervous System: There have been rare reports consistent with, but not diagnostic of, extrapyramidal reactions in patients receiving ondansetron.

Cardiovascular: Rare instances of tachycardia, angina (chest pain), bradycardia, hypotension, syncope, and electrocardiographic alterations, including second degree heart block. In many cases the relationship to Zofran Injection was unclear.

Special Senses: Transient blurred vision, in some cases associated with abnormalities of accommodation, and transient dizziness during or shortly after IV infusion.

Local Reactions: Pain, redness, and burning at site of injection.

Other: Rare cases of hypokalemia and grand mal seizures have been reported. The relationship to Zofran Injection was unclear. Rare cases of hypersensitivity reactions, sometimes severe (e.g., anaphylaxis, bronchospasm, shortness of breath, hypotension, shock, angioedema, urticaria), have also been reported.

Postoperative Nausea and Vomiting: The following adverse events have been reported in $\geq 2\%$ of people receiving ondansetron at a dosage of 4 mg IV over 2 to 5 minutes in clinical trials. Rates of these events were not significantly different in the ondansetron and placebo groups. These patients were receiving multiple concomitant perioperative and postoperative medications.

	Zofran Injection 4 mg IV n=547 patients	Placebo n=547 patients
Headache	92 (17%)	77 (14%)
Dizziness	67 (12%)	88 (16%)
Musculoskeletal pain	57 (10%)	59 (11%)
Drowsiness/sedation	44 (8%)	37 (7%)
Shivers	38 (7%)	39 (7%)
Malaise/fatigue	25 (5%)	30 (5%)
Injection site reaction	21 (4%)	18 (3%)
Urinary retention	17 (3%)	15 (3%)
Postoperative CO_2-related pain*	12 (2%)	16 (3%)
Chest pain (unspecified)	12 (2%)	15 (3%)
Anxiety/agitation	11 (2%)	16 (3%)
Dysuria	11 (2%)	9 (2%)
Hypotension	10 (2%)	12 (2%)
Fever	10 (2%)	6 (1%)
Cold sensation	9 (2%)	8 (1%)
Pruritus	9 (2%)	3 (<1%)
Paresthesia	9 (2%)	2 (<1%)

*Sites of pain included abdomen, stomach, joints, rib cage, shoulder.

Drug Abuse and Dependence: Animal studies have shown that ondansetron is not discriminated as a benzodiazepine nor does it substitute for benzodiazepines in direct addiction studies.

Zofran® (ondansetron hydrochloride) Injection

OVERDOSAGE: There is no specific antidote for ondansetron overdose. Patients should be managed with appropriate supportive therapy. Individual doses as large as 145 mg and total daily dosages (three doses) as large as 252 mg have been administered intravenously without significant adverse events. These doses are more than 10 times the recommended daily dose.

"Sudden blindness" (amaurosis) of 2 to 3 minutes' duration plus severe constipation occurred in one patient that was administered 72 mg of ondansetron intravenously as a single dose. Hypotension (and faintness) occurred in another patient that took 48 mg of oral ondansetron. Following infusion of 32 mg over only a 4-minute period, a vasovagal episode with transient second degree heart block was observed. In all instances, the events resolved completely.

DOSAGE AND ADMINISTRATION:
Cancer Chemotherapy: DILUTE BEFORE USE. Zofran® Injection should be diluted in 50 mL of 5% dextrose injection or 0.9% sodium chloride injection before administration. The recommended IV dosage of Zofran Injection is a single 32-mg dose or three 0.15-mg/kg doses. A single 32-mg dose is infused over 15 minutes beginning 30 minutes before the start of emetogenic chemotherapy. The recommended infusion rate should not be exceeded (see OVERDOSAGE). With the three-dose (0.15-mg/kg) regimen, the first dose is infused over 15 minutes beginning 30 minutes before the start of emetogenic chemotherapy. Subsequent doses (0.15 mg/kg) are administered 4 and 8 hours after the first dose of Zofran Injection.

Zofran Injection should not be mixed with solutions for which physical and chemical compatibility have not been established. In particular, this applies to alkaline solutions as a precipitate may form.

Pediatric Use: **DILUTE BEFORE USE.** On the basis of the limited available information (see CLINICAL TRIALS: Pediatric Studies and CLINICAL PHARMACOLOGY: Pharmacokinetics), the dosage in children 4 to 18 years of age should be three 0.15-mg/kg doses (see above). Little information is available about dosage in children 3 years of age or younger.

Use in the Elderly: **DILUTE BEFORE USE.** The dosage is the same as for the general population.
Prevention of Postoperative Nausea and/or Vomiting: NO DILUTION NECESSARY. Immediately before induction of anesthesia, or postoperatively if the patient experiences nausea and/or vomiting occurring shortly after surgery, administer 4 mg **undiluted** intravenously in not less than 30 seconds, preferably over 2 to 5 minutes. Repeat dosing for patients who continue to experience nausea and/or vomiting postoperatively has not been studied. While recommended as a fixed dose for all, few patients above 80 kg or below 40 kg have been studied.

Pediatric Use: There is no experience with the use of Zofran Injection in the prevention or treatment of postoperative nausea and vomiting in children.

Use in the Elderly: **NO DILUTION NECESSARY.** The dosage recommendation is the same as for the general population.
Dosage Adjustment for Patients With Impaired Renal Function: No specific studies have been conducted in patients with renal insufficiency.
Dosage Adjustment for Patients With Impaired Hepatic Function: In patients with severe hepatic impairment according to Child-Pugh[1] criteria, a single maximal daily dose of 8 mg to be infused over 15 minutes beginning 30 minutes before the start of the emetogenic chemotherapy is recommended. There is no experience beyond first-day administration of ondansetron.
Stability: Zofran Injection is stable at room temperature under normal lighting conditions for 48 hours after dilution with the following IV fluids: 0.9% sodium chloride injection, 5% dextrose injection, 5% dextrose and 0.9% sodium chloride injection, 5% dextrose and 0.45% sodium chloride injection, and 3% sodium chloride injection.

Although Zofran Injection is chemically and physically stable when diluted as recommended, sterile precautions should be observed because diluents generally do not contain preservative. After dilution, do not use beyond 24 hours.
Note: Parenteral drug products should be inspected visually for particulate matter and discoloration before administration whenever solution and container permit.

Zofran® (ondansetron hydrochloride) Injection

Precaution: Occasionally, ondansetron precipitates at the stopper/vial interface in vials stored upright. Potency and safety are not affected. If a precipitate is observed, resolubilize by shaking the vial vigorously.

HOW SUPPLIED: Zofran® Injection, 2 mg/mL, is supplied in 2-mL single-dose vials (NDC 0173-0442-0) and in 20-mL multidose vials (NDC 0173-0442-00).
  Store between 2° and 30°C (36° and 86°F). Protect from light.

REFERENCE: 1. Pugh RNH, Murray-Lyon IM, Dawson JL, Pietroni MC, Williams R. Transection of the oesophagus for bleeding oesophageal varices. *Br J Surg.* 1973;60:646-649.

CERENEX™

PHARMACEUTICALS
DIVISION OF GLAXO INC.
Research Triangle Park, NC 27709

April 199
RL-10

Reference:
1. Complete Prescribing Information, ZOFRAN® (ondansetron HCl) Injection. April 1994.